C. STRACHAN
7 Queens Road,
Dovercourt,
Harwich, Essex,
CO12 3TH
Tel. 0255 506420

Surgical Dermatology

David J. Eedy

MD MRCP
Consultant Dermatologist
Craigavon Area Hospital Group Trust
Craigavon, Northern Ireland, UK

Stephen M. Breathnach

MA MD PhD FRCP
Consultant Dermatologist and Senior Lecturer
St John's Institute of Dermatology
St Thomas' Hospital, London, UK
Consultant Dermatologist
Epsom Healthcare NHS Trust, Epsom, UK

Neil P.J. Walker

BSc FRCP
Honorary Consultant Dermatologist
The Oxford Radcliffe Hospital, Oxford, UK

Blackwell
Science

To our families and colleagues

© 1996 by
Blackwell Science Ltd
Editorial Offices:
Osney Mead, Oxford OX2 0EL
25 John Street, London WC1N 2BL
23 Ainslie Place, Edinburgh EH3 6AJ
238 Main Street, Cambridge
  Massachusetts 02142, USA
54 University Street, Carlton
  Victoria 3053, Australia

Other Editorial Offices:
Arnette Blackwell SA
  224, Boulevard Saint Germain
  75007 Paris, France

Blackwell Wissenschafts-Verlag GmbH
  Kurfürstendamm 57
  10707 Berlin, Germany

  Zehetnergasse 6
  A-1140 Wien
  Austria

First published 1996

Set by Excel Typesetters
Company, Hong Kong
Printed and bound in Italy
by Rotolito Lombarda S.p.A., Milan

The Blackwell Science logo is a
trade mark of Blackwell Science Ltd,
registered at the United Kingdom
Trade Marks Registry

DISTRIBUTORS

Marston Book Services Ltd
PO Box 269
Abingdon
Oxon OX14 4YN
(*Orders*: Tel: 01235 465500
           Fax: 01235 465555)

USA
Blackwell Science, Inc.
238 Main Street
Cambridge, MA 02142
(*Orders*: Tel: 800 215-1000
           617 876-7000
           Fax: 617 492-5263)

Canada
Copp Clark, Ltd
2775 Matheson Blvd East
Mississauga, Ontario
Canada, L4W 4P7
(*Orders*: Tel: 800 263-4374
           905 238-6074)

Australia
Blackwell Science Pty Ltd
54 University Street
Carlton, Victoria 3053
(*Orders*: Tel: 03 9347 0300
           Fax: 03 9349 3016)

A catalogue record for this title
is available from the British Library

ISBN 0-632-03425-4

Library of Congress
Cataloging-in-publication Data

Eedy, David J.
    Surgical dermatology/David J.
Eedy, Stephen M. Breathnach, and
Neil P.J. Walker.
        p.   cm.
    Includes bibliographical references
and index.
    ISBN 0-632-03425-4
    1. Skin—Surgery.
I. Breathnach, Stephen M.
II. Walker, Neil P.J.   III. Title.
    [DNLM: 1 Skin Diseases—surgery.
WR 140 E26s   1996]
RD520.E44   1996
617.4'77—dc20
DNLM/DLC
for Library of Congress   95-52144
                                        CIP

Contents

Preface

Traditionally, dermatology has always had recourse to a significant body of surgical techniques. However, recent years have seen a substantial growth in the development and use of such procedures, both in response to the increase in skin cancer and patient demand for aesthetic procedures. As a result, surgical dermatology has increasingly become a recognised sub-specialty, growing ever more popular with both hospital departments and patients.

The basic principles of dermatological surgery addressed in this book refer to the application of these skills, whether at the level of primary care physician, outpatient surgical clinic, or at the level of the hospital dermatology department. Access to such skills is, therefore, recognised as having a significant place in the repertoire of a wide range of physicians, giving rise to the need for a textbook of broad appeal. Throughout the book we have tried to illustrate and explain the techniques involved in the hope that a clear understanding of the underlying principles will result in good surgical practice.

The book does not aim to be an exhaustive description of all the techniques currently available to the modern dermatological surgeon. With this in mind a list of useful references is given at the end of each chapter. These give prominence to review articles on each subject, or keynote articles that give the reader a potential starting point for those wishing to peruse the subject in greater depth.

We wish to acknowledge with gratitude the many colleagues, either through informal discussion or encouragement, who have helped in the evolution of the manuscript. Where colleagues have given clinical photographs for use in the book, their permission has been sought, and acknowledgement is made in the text. We also wish to acknowledge Mr Stuart Robertson, Department of Illustration, St John's Institute of Dermatology and Miss H Smith, Department of Medical Photography, Craigavon Area Hospital Group Trust, without whose help and professional skills we would have been unable to provide the extensive photographic illustrations. We would also wish to acknowledge the invaluable help of Debbie Maizels who produced the line artwork used throughout the book. Finally, we wish to thank those at Blackwell Science, and in particular Stuart Taylor and Lorna Dickson, for their forbearance, advice and help at all stages of the production process.

David J. Eedy
Stephen M. Breathnach
Neil P.J. Walker

1 Equipping the theatre

Most dermatological surgery is performed in an outpatient setting, and so the correct design for the dermatological outpatient theatre is of paramount importance. The size of the room itself will depend on the operator's preference and on the facilities available. However, for comfort in performing cutaneous surgery, the dimensions should be at least 3 m × 4.3 m, since smaller rooms become cramped when they have to accommodate the patient, the surgeon and an assistant, as well as equipment and trolleys. Doors need to be wide enough to allow patients to be moved from the theatre on a stretcher in the event of an emergency. Cabinets to contain instruments, dressings, anaesthetics and sterile supplies, and a readily accessible emergency box for resuscitation, are essential, and should have an acrylic or formica finish. A separate area for washing and scrubbing hands is preferable. Ideally, the theatre floor should be covered with tiles or linoleum, and the walls with vinyl or tiling, for ease of cleaning.

1.1 The operating table

One of the most important items of equipment for both the convenience of the surgeon and the comfort of the patient is the operating table, the height of which should be easily adjustable to allow the surgeon to work equally well in either the sitting or standing position (Fig. 1.1). The table should be fitted with hinged joints to enable elevation at the head and/or back and at the foot, as well as having a tilt facility for easy assumption of the head-down (Trendelenburg's) position in case of an emergency. There should be a detachable side extension to support an outstretched arm, as for hand or nail surgery. A proper degree of padding contributes substantially to the comfort of the patient. While this specially designed type of table is the ideal, many surgeons may have to make do with the considerably less optimal alternative of an ordinary examination couch. Whichever type of table is used, it should be placed so that the surgeon has adequate space to approach the patient from either side.

1.2 Lighting equipment

Adequate illumination of the operating field is vital during dermatological surgery. The choice among the wide variety of lighting units on the market will depend on available funds. Ceiling-mounted lights are the most versatile and convenient, since they are readily adjustable by handles which may be sterilised, allowing the surgeon to manipulate the lighting during a procedure. A good option is the diffused central, ceiling-mounted, cool, high-intensity beam light (Illuminator 4®), which is easily adjusted and gives a high intensity light (Fig. 1.2). This design eliminates shadows, and

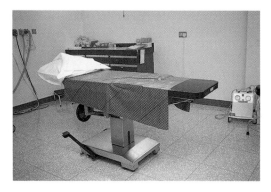

Fig. 1.1 Operating table with adjustable head support height and table height.

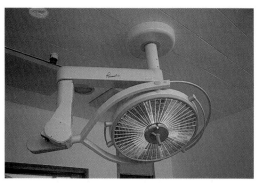

Fig. 1.2 Adjustable ceiling-mounted high-intensity beam light.

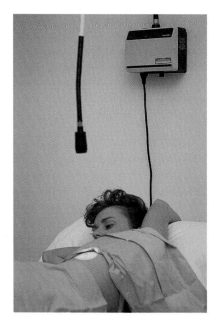

Fig. 1.3 Adjustable fibre-optic wall-mounted light source.

arm pivot points provide unlimited rotation. An adequate option comprises four outer-focusable bulbs and a central pre-focused bulb, or the cheaper option of a single ceiling-mounted focusable light.

Free-standing mobile pedestal lighting units (Derungs®, Waldmann Lichttechnik®) can be obtained, but have the disadvantage that they take up valuable floor space and obstruct movement around the table. Wall-mounted lights are less versatile, and necessitate the operating table being placed against a wall, thus restricting free access to the patient from both sides. However, a useful form of wall-mounted light is the flexible, fibre-optic light (Halogen Bright Spot®) which delivers a focusable source of light (Fig. 1.3), and which comes with disposable sterile sheaths, allowing movement of the beam in any direction during surgery by an operator. Less adaptable are a variety of wall or stand-based examination lamps with telescopic and pivoted arms.

1.3 Instrument stand

The most commonly used form of instrument stand is a stainless steel dressing trolley, fitted with non-static castors. It usually has two shelves, the upper of which acts as a tray for supporting instruments in use on a sterile towel; the lower can be used as a temporary storage space for miscellaneous items needed during surgery, such as antiseptic solutions. Some are available with drawers beneath the top shelf where sterile instruments can also be stored. The advantage of such a trolley is the ease with which it can be wheeled around the operating theatre, should the surgeon require to move during the procedure. An alternative, but more expensive, option is the Mayo stand; this incorporates a mobile support which, when wheeled under the operating table, positions the tray of the instrument stand over the patient's body without resting on it. Also available are autoclavable reusable instrument mats, which can be placed on a sterile towel laid on the patient; these have grooves for holding instruments in place, enabling rapid retrieval of instruments adjacent to the operating field.

1.4 Disposal of waste

In order to provide a clear field for the surgeon, and to ensure control of contaminated material, it is essential to establish a procedure for disposal of blood-soaked swabs. Use of a mobile open-top stainless steel wastebucket on castors provides a convenient solution.

1.5 Instruments for dermatological surgery

Scalpel holders and blades

By far the most frequently used scalpel handle is the standard Bard–Parker No. 3 autoclavable steel handle (Fig. 1.4), which may be ordered with or without an imprinted ruler on the scalpel handle; the latter is especially useful for measuring the size of lesions and for the planning of flaps. Other variations include a heavier round No. 3 handle, and the slimmer No. 7 handle (Fig. 1.4).

Scalpel blades in common use are made of carbon steel (Fig. 1.5). For the Bard–Parker handle, the No. 15 blade is suitable for most dermatological

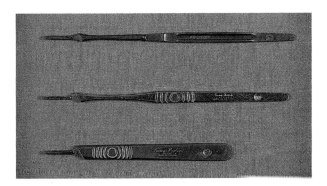

Fig. 1.4 Scalpel handles. From top to bottom, No. 7, No. 5, No. 3.

surgery; the blade is sharpest at its belly, and therefore cutting should be done with this part of the blade rather than the tip. Another useful blade is the No. 11 blade which has a pointed tip for stab incisions, such as in draining abscesses, or for suture removal. The No. 10 blade is large and rounded and is designed for larger excisions, for example on the back; it is also useful for performing shave excisions or biopsies.

The Beaver scalpel handle, which has a hexagonal cross-section for ease of grip and manipulation, is useful for delicate work. A selection of special scalpel blades are available for this instrument; the No. 67 blade is equivalent to the standard No. 15 Bard–Parker blade.

The double-edged Gillette®, Jewel® or Wilkinson Sword® razor-blade, when broken in half (Fig. 1.6), is well suited for shave excision.

Sterile disposable plastic scalpel holders with pre-attached blades of standard sizes (Fig. 1.7), are an alternative to reusable steel scalpel handles; they have the obvious advantage of not requiring autoclaving, and are easily disposed of following a surgical procedure. Disposable scalpel holders with a sheath (Personna Safety Scalpel®), which can be advanced to cover the blade following use give added protection against accidental injury (Fig. 1.8a,b).

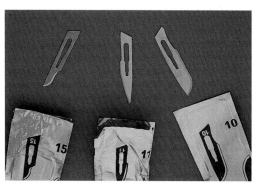

Fig. 1.5 Scalpel blades most commonly used.

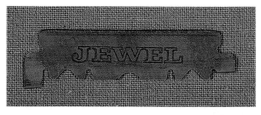

Fig. 1.6 Razor-blade broken in half for shave excision.

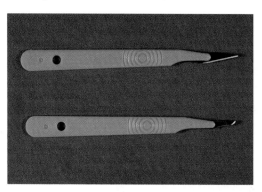

Fig. 1.7 Disposable scalpels. From top to bottom, No. 11, No. 15.

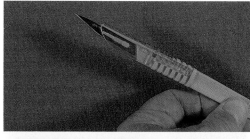

a

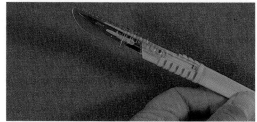

b

Fig. 1.8 Personna Safety Scalpel® **a** With sheath retracted and **b**, with sheath advanced.

Blade removers

Simple blade extractors, which reduce the chances of accidental injury, can be obtained to remove blades from No. 3 or No. 7 handles quickly and safely. A more sophisticated scalpel blade remover is shown in Fig. 1.9.

Forceps

Swab/sponge forceps

Some operators prefer to use swab or sponge forceps for cleansing the patient's skin. These have the advantage that the operator's gloves do not become contaminated with skin organisms during the skin cleansing process, but they are an option rather than a necessity (Fig. 1.10).

Tissue-handling forceps

These are available with and without teeth. Toothed forceps are preferable for tissue handling, since they allow tissue to be held firmly despite only light pressure between the tips of the forceps, resulting in less tissue damage. The most widely used general purpose forceps is the Adson type (Fig. 1.11a,b). The standard tip size is 1 mm, but finer tips are available.

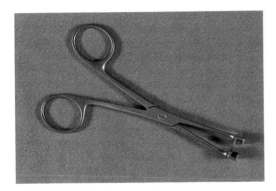

Fig. 1.9 Tiemann® scalpel blade remover.

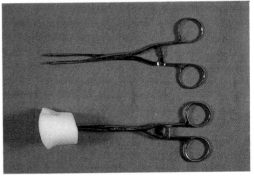

Fig. 1.10 Sponge forceps with serrated tips.

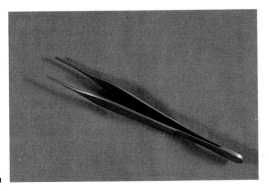

a

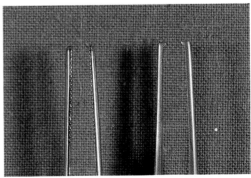

b

Fig. 1.11 a. Adson's (dural) forceps; **b.** (left) serrated forceps; (right) toothed.

5

Non-toothed Adson's forceps with a serrated tip (Fig. 1.11b), must be handled gently to avoid tissue crush injury and a poor cosmetic result. Iris forceps available with either a serrated or a toothed tip are suitable for delicate work, for example around the eyelid where the skin is particularly thin.

Artery forceps

The most frequently used artery forceps in dermatological surgery is the Halsted's Mosquito artery forceps, available with either a straight or a curved tip (Fig. 1.12). Probably the most versatile is the 5 in straight-tipped forceps, although the curved tip version is invaluable for reaching bleeding vessels in areas of undermining.

Scissors

A wide variety of types of scissors is available (Fig. 1.13), and it is important to realise that each is designed for a specific purpose, and may not be appropriate for a different task. For example, scissors designed for undermining, or for cutting delicate skin tissue, should never be used for suture cutting, as this will very significantly reduce the life span of the instrument.

Tissue-cutting scissors

Cutting scissors can usually be obtained in either a straight blade or a curved blade version (Fig. 1.14). Straight scissors provide more precise straight-line cutting, whereas curved scissors may be useful in awkward sites, as well as for cutting skin tags etc. Perhaps the most versatile scissors is the cradle scissors, which is relatively strong and useful for general work. For delicate work, as on the face and around the eyelids, iris scissors (Fig. 1.13) are invaluable.

Undermining scissors

Dissecting and undermining scissors should be blunt tipped (Fig. 1.15).
Cradle or Stephen's Tenotomy scissors with blunt tips can be used for

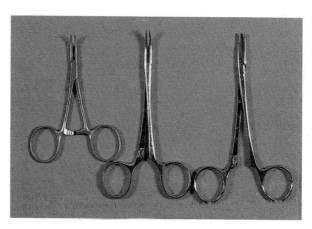

Fig. 1.12 Artery forceps. (Left and centre) curved tipped; (right) straight.

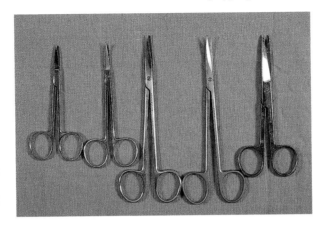

Fig. 1.13 Some commonly used scissors. (From left to right) iris scissors (straight), iris scissors (curved), Aufricht scissors (straight), Aufricht scissors (curved) and suture-cutting scissors.

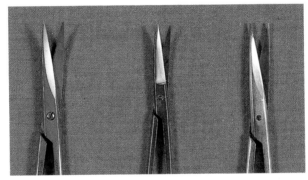

Fig. 1.14 Sharp-pointed tissue-cutting scissors.

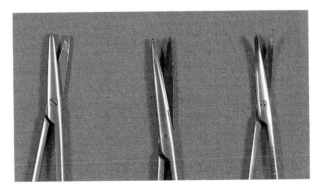

Fig. 1.15 Blunt-tipped tissue-dissecting scissors.

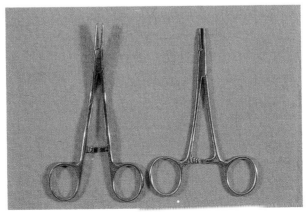

Fig. 1.16 Needle holders with serrated jaws.

undermining as well as for cutting tissue; the curved versions help to keep the plane of undermining parallel to the skin surface. Metzenbaum scissors with blunt tips, available in straight or curved versions, are ideal for undermining more extensive areas in tough tissue sites such as the central back.

Dressing scissors

The Lister bandage scissors, with angulated blades and a large blunt tip, slip between the bandage and the skin without risk of skin damage, and are ideal for bandage removal. However, any other heavy duty scissors with a blunt tip are adequate for this type of procedure.

Needle holders

The choice among the large variety of needle holders available will depend on operator preference and the delicacy of the procedure to be carried out. Needle holders are available with serrated or smooth jaws (Fig. 1.16); smooth jaws are useful for small needle sizes, while cross-serrated tips ensure a more secure grasp on the suture or needle, but may cause fraying of braided sutures or damage to the needle itself. Perhaps the most versatile is the Webster 5 in needle holder, with another alternative being the Halsey 4.75 in or 5 in needle holder; both are available with either smooth or serrated jaws. The sturdy Crile Murray's needle holder can be used with larger needles when operating on the back or scalp. The Castroviejo needle holder (Fig. 1.17), which has very small tips and opens with a spring action, is useful for placing very small sutures in delicate work, as on the face; again, they can be obtained with either smooth or serrated jaws.

Skin hooks

Skin hooks (Fig. 1.18) have the advantage over forceps for atraumatic handling of skin during undermining and placement of sutures, in that they do not crush tissue, and therefore produce a better cosmetic result. Examples include the Gillies skin hook, or the somewhat larger Fraser 5 in skin hook, with a single point which may be either sharp or blunt (Fig. 1.18). Some operators prefer versions with multiple prongs, such as the Lehey skin hook, which may have less tendency to tear tissue.

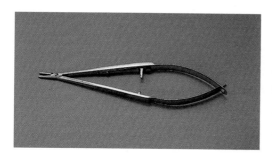

Fig. 1.17 Castroviejo needle holder.

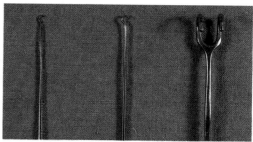

Fig. 1.18 Gillies skin hooks and Lehey skin hook.

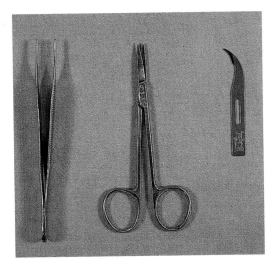

Fig. 1.19 Adson's forceps (non-toothed) and fine scissors for suture removal. Suture removal blade (right).

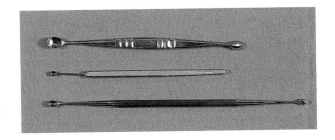

Fig. 1.20 Oval dermal curettes of varying size.

Suture removal

A standard suture removal set is illustrated in Fig. 1.19.

Adson's forceps can be used for most suture removal, but epilating forceps (e.g. Whitfield's forceps) which may be straight, curved or angled, are sometimes preferable.

Suture removal requires a sturdy form of scissors, such as the Spencer scissors which have a notch at the tip into which the suture can be placed. For extra-fine suture removal, Iris Bonn micro-forceps are suitable. Disposable suture removal scissors (Steriseal®) designed for once-only use are also available, but these tend to be rather coarse.

Cheaper alternatives to specially designed scissors for suture removal include the use of a No. 11 blade without a handle, and stitch cutter blades with a curved tip.

Curettes

One of the most frequently used instruments in office practice is the dermal curette. Curettes are available in a variety of sizes, and in either open or closed-head versions. Closed-head curettes may have oval or round heads, and cup sizes range from 1 to 6 mm (Fig. 1.20). A typical example is the Exner curette, which has round and oval heads at opposite ends of the instrument. The Volkmann spoon curette may be used to remove larger

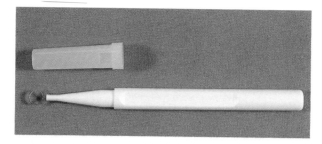

Fig. 1.21 Disposable ring curette.

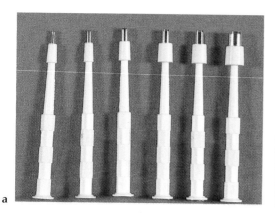

a

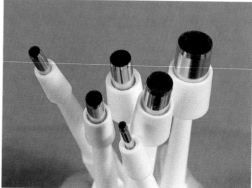

b

Fig. 1.22 a. Range of disposable punches and **b**. cutting edge of punches.

lesions. Open-headed disposable curettes are also available (Fig. 1.21), and have the advantages of always being sharp, coming in a variety of sizes and in sterile sealed packages ready for use (Stiefel®), but are an expensive option for those who use curettes on a regular basis.

Disposable punches

Punches used for biopsies of skin are usually of the once-only use disposable type with a plastic handle, and are available in sizes of 2, 3, 4, 5, 6 and 8 mm (Stiefel®) (Fig. 1.22a,b), and with an oval cutting edge in sizes of 3 × 7.5 mm and 4 × 8 mm (Acu-E-Punch®). These have the advantage of not requiring sharpening or sterilisation before use. Reusable Keyes punches (Fig. 1.23), may be preferred by some surgeons, especially for hair transplantation work.

1.6 Sterile drapes and towel clips

Sterile drapes, which protect the field of surgery from bacteria, are essential for the maintenance of wound sterility, and may be either of the disposable or non-disposable type. Non-disposable cloth drapes, which can be washed, autoclaved and reused, are ideal if a central sterile supply unit is available, and have the advantage of being comfortable for the patient. They are best

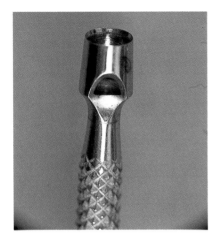
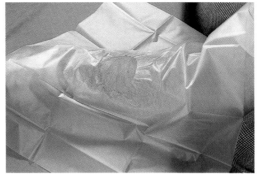

Fig. 1.23 Keyes punch.   **Fig. 1.24** Disposable Steri-drape®.

held securely in place using sterile clips such as the Backhaus towel clip or the Mayo forceps, although artery forceps can be used. Disposable paper drapes are cheap, but are difficult to control during the operation, and when wet with blood tend to lose their barrier function against infection. A better but more expensive alternative is the use of a disposable plastic drape (Fig. 1.24) with a central opening (Steri-drape®), which is held to the skin surrounding the wound by adhesive tape. This drape has the advantages of being easy to control and impermeable to blood and bacteria, although it may be less suitable for surgery around the nose and mouth.

1.7 Cotton gauze and buds

Cotton gauze is made in eight types, type 1 being the tightest woven gauze while type 8 is the least tightly woven. It is also described in terms of its ply; this being the number of layers present after the gauze has been folded to its final shape. The ply is most commonly 8, 12 or 16 ply. Clearly, the greater the ply the greater will be its capacity for absorption of blood at the time of surgery. Gauze may also be categorised according to its folded size, this usually being 2 × 2 in, 3 × 3 in or 4 × 4 in. Some types of gauze incorporate an X-ray opaque line through it, enabling detection on subsequent X-ray in case of inadvertent failure to remove it from a body cavity. Sterile cotton buds (Fig. 1.25) are useful for controlling small areas of bleeding and for the application of haemostatic agents and antibiotic preparations.

1.8 Autoclaves

It is clearly essential that all instruments used for surgery are autoclaved prior to use, to avoid not only bacterial infection but also the risk of transmission of hepatitis B and human immunodeficiency virus (HIV). There are a variety of autoclaves of different sizes and prices, which comply fully with the British Standards specifications, available to practitioners who do not have access to a hospital's Central Sterile Supply Department. One widely

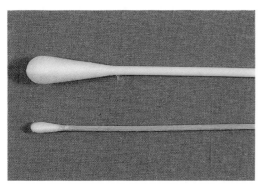

Fig. 1.25 Cotton buds suitable for autoclaving.

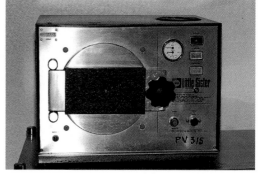

Fig. 1.26 Little Sister® autoclave.

used autoclave is the Little Sister® 3 model, with an operating temperature of 134°C, a drying cycle and comprehensive safety features to prevent over-heating (Fig. 1.26). The three removable shelves are more than adequate to accommodate the instruments a dermatologist may contemplate using. A similar device is the Eschmann 2000® autoclave (SES 2000), which also offers the option of sterilising with or without a drying cycle, and gives an audible and visual signal at the completion of the cycle. A rather cheaper autoclave, in which instruments are placed standing in the drum of the machine, is produced by Prestige Medical®. The sterilising cycle of this device is set at 126°C, and the time for sterilisation is consequently a little longer. This type of autoclave does not have a drying sequence at the end of the autoclaving cycle, so that if instruments are required in the dry state they must be placed in sealed pouches prior to autoclaving.

1.9 Cautery equipment

Cautery is one of the best established methods for the control of bleeding and for induction of tissue necrosis, and works on the principle that electrical resistance to the passage of direct current through a wire circuit results in the generation of heat. Cautery has the advantage of giving good haemostasis even in the presence of blood in the field, but associated tissue damage may lead to impaired wound healing and a compromised cosmetic result.

A standard device is illustrated in Fig. 1.27. The heat output of the device may be adjusted by a knob attached to a rheostat within the cautery control box. Interchangeable reusable, sterilisable tips used for cautery range from the small ball or sharp tip variety suitable for vessel coagulation or lesion destruction, to the flat expanded variety designed for cutting through the base of lesions such as skin papillomata.

Hand-held rechargeable cautery units have recently become available (Fig. 1.28). These come equipped with a variety of reusable tips which are easily transported in a flat case, and a lightweight handle which can be carried in a pocket or bag. The handle contains rechargeable batteries, which when fully charged can provide up to 15 min of heat output, or approximately 300 3 s bursts of heat. Although convenient, they cannot compete with the heavy duty alternatives where substantial power output

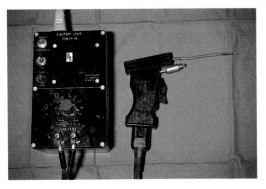

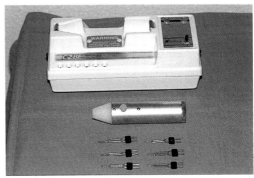

Fig. 1.27 Typical cautery box with rheostat control and cautery unit.

Fig. 1.28 Hand-held rechargeable cautery unit.

is necessary. Recently, a disposable, hand-held, battery-operated cautery unit has been developed (Aaron®), which has similar characteristics to the rechargeable units.

Electrosurgical units

A number of versatile electrosurgical devices exist (the Ellman Surgitron®, Fig. 1.29; Martin Mini 40D®, Martin ME® 50 and 80 which afford a selection of output modes, providing a choice between microcoagulation, cutting and coagulation, haemostasis and desiccation/fulguration. A host of different reusable tips for specific indications is available in either unipolar (Fig. 1.30) or bipolar mode (Fig. 1.31). A disadvantage is that use of these devices is accompanied by a more than usually prominent burning smell and smoke plume. The problem can be overcome by an exhaust extractor (Fig. 1.32), but this adds substantially to the cost of the device.

Hyfrecator

A hyfrecator is an electrical surgical device which generates current for desiccation or coagulation, but does not have the facility for cutting. The

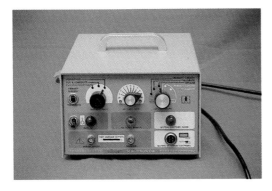

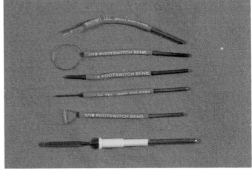

Fig. 1.29 Ellman® electrosurgical unit for unipolar and bipolar modes.

Fig. 1.30 Range of unipolar tips for electrosurgical unit.

13

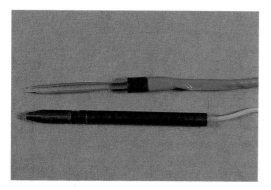

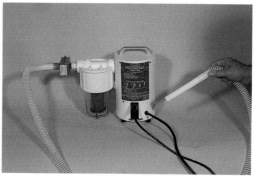

Fig. 1.31 Bipolar forceps (top). Unipolar handle (bottom).

Fig. 1.32 Smoke evacuator unit.

surgeon has the option of choosing between monopolar and bipolar output modes from the device. The monopolar output provides a high-frequency, high-voltage current discharge from one electrode tip to the patient, whereas the bipolar mode provides a high-frequency current which travels back and forth between the two terminals (usually the tips of forceps) of the device, ensuring excellent coagulation. One disadvantage of the hyfrecator is that it requires a relatively dry field to work efficiently. Hyfrecators can be activated either using a foot switch or via a switch on the hyfrecator handle. Both sterile disposable and reusable electrode tips are available for use in the monopolar mode, while for the bipolar mode a variety of autoclavable forceps, including the Adson-type forceps, can be obtained.

The most widely used hyfrecator is the Birtcher® hyfrecator. The power output control on the 733 model, now being phased out, is a rotating knob on the front of the control box of the machine. Power output from the new Birtcher Hyfrecator Plus® (7-796 model, Fig. 1.33) is displayed digitally, and can be adjusted via controls on the handle or on the box.

1.10 Suction

A suction unit should be available for anything but the most basic surgery, to allow good visualisation of the surgical field. In a hospital setting, wall suction may be provided. Alternatively, small portable units, to which pre-sterilised suction tubing can be attached, may be obtained. Examples include the 3 A Suction pump®, Vacu-Aide® and De Vilbiss® pumps.

1.11 Syringes and needles

A variety of plastic sterile disposable syringes (1 ml, 5 ml, 10 ml and 12 ml) should be available. Syringes with a luer lock, which prevents needle detachment during administration of local anaesthetic, are useful. A useful range of needles is illustrated in Fig. 1.34. Some surgeons prefer a dental syringe specifically designed to accept disposable local anaesthetic cartridges, equipped with fine disposable needles. Sterile 1 ml disposable

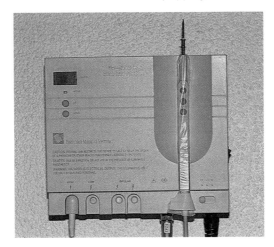

Fig. 1.33 Birtcher® hyfrecator with electronic control.

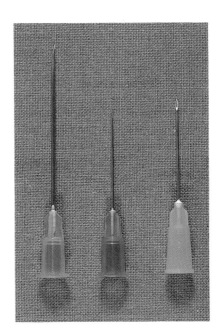

Fig. 1.34 Commonly used needles: gauges 25 (left), 21 (middle) and 23 (right).

syringes with an integral fine needle (Microfine® insulin syringe) may also be useful.

1.12 A basic skin surgery tray

A basic skin surgery tray will usually be chosen by each surgeon to suit individual needs. A suggested skin surgery tray that will probably suit the needs of most surgeons performing regular skin surgery is shown in Figs 1.35 and 1.36 and contains the following items.

Scalpel blade holder
Halsey needle holder × 1
Aufricht dissecting scissors (straight) × 1
Aufricht dissecting scissors (curved) × 1

15

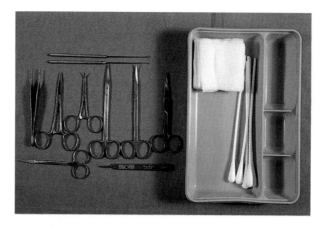

Fig. 1.35 Simple basic skin surgery tray suitable for most purposes.

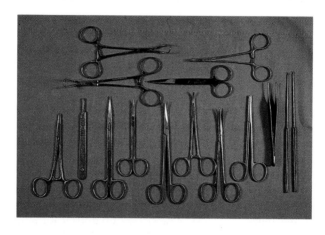

Fig. 1.36 Range of surgical instruments for ideal skin surgery tray.

Metzenbaum scissors with blunt tips (straight) × 1
Metzenbaum scissors with blunt tips (curved) × 1
Gillies fine skin hooks × 2
Iris scissors (curved) × 1
Mosquito forceps (curved) × 2
Adson dural forceps (toothed) × 1
Backhaus towel clips (5 in) × 2
Set-up tray (moulded plastic, subdivided into compartments, auto-
    clavable) × 1
Sterile gauze 3 × 3 in (8 ply)
Sterile surgical drapes (× 2)
Cotton buds

1.13 Resuscitation equipment

Emergencies in dermatological surgery are thankfully rare, but it is nevertheless mandatory to have ready access to adequate resuscitation equipment and emergency drugs. In addition, staff should be trained in
cardiopulmonary resuscitation and preferably attend regular refresher
courses, to ensure that a patient at risk can be stabilised and transferred to
an emergency care facility as quickly as possible.

A stethoscope and sphygomanometer are basic items of equipment. An airway is an essential part of any emergency pack. This may be of the standard curved type, designed to fit behind the tongue, but a new type produced by Vitalograph® combines the traditional curved piece for the oral route with an attachment to allow nasal ventilation. An Ambu-bag® for ventilation is another very important piece of resuscitation equipment; a suitable variety is the Vitalograph® reusable bag, which comes fitted with an adult cupped mask. A variety of kits is available which include the above items with a laryngoscope. A portable suction device is a further necessity; the Vitalograph® emergency aspirator, with hand-operated suction which will work in any orientation, is particularly useful. The amount of equipment obtained will depend on the complexity of the operative procedures carried out; for those embarking on more extensive procedures such as deep chemical peels, a cardiac monitor and a defibrillator will be required.

Emergency resuscitation drugs should be stored, usually in ampoule form, so that they are immediately accessible in case of a cardiovascular emergency. Needles, syringes and intravenous cannulae must be close at hand. It is vital that the surgeon and assisting staff know where the resuscitation equipment and drugs are stored, and how they should be used. The telephone number of the local cardiac crash call team should be displayed in a prominent place, to enable its swift response to provide back-up when the patient's condition has been stabilised.

Emergency drugs

A variety of drugs will be required to cover all eventualities in the case of an emergency. The emergency drug box should be checked regularly for drug expiry and to ensure that any used items have been replaced.

The following drugs, while not an exhaustive list, should provide for the vast majority of emergencies.

Emergency drugs for dermatological surgery

Cardiorespiratory drugs and diuretics (injections)

Aminophylline 250 mg/10 ml (2 ampoules)
Adrenaline 1:1000 (1 ml) (2 ampoules)
Adrenaline 1:10 000 (0.1 mg/ml) in 10 ml syringe with intracardiac needles (×2)
Atropine 0.6 mg/ml (2 ampoules)
Lignocaine 5% 10 ml vial (2 syringes)
Sodium bicarbonate 4.2% 10 ml (disposable syringe) (4 syringes)
Calcium chloride 10% in 10 ml (2 ampoules)
Frusemide 20 mg/2 ml or bumetanide 1 mg/4 ml (2 ampoules)
Diazoxide 300 mg/20 ml × 1
Propranolol 1 mg/ml or labetalol 100 mg/20 ml
Water for injection 10 ml (×4) (2 ampoules)
Metaraminol 10 mg/1 ml *or* noradrenaline 0.2 mg/2 ml (2 ampoules)

Transfusion sets with packs (each 500 mg × 2) of:
    saline 0.9%;
    dextrose 5%;
    sodium bicarbonate 1.4%; and
    plasma expanders, for example Dextran 70® or Haemacel®.

Oral cardiorespiratory
    Glyceryl trinitrate 300 µg tablets or glyceryl trinitrate spray 400 µg per
        metered dose
    Nifedipine 5 mg capsules

Allergic reactions
    Dexamethasone 4 mg/2 ml (× 2) (2 ampoules)
    Hydrocortisone sodium succinate 500 mg
    Chlorpheniramine 10 mg/ml (2 ampoules)
    Aminophylline and adrenaline (as above)

Anti-convulsants/sedatives
    Diazepam 10 mg/2 ml (2 ampoules)
    Diabetics:
        soluble insulin 100 U/ml (1 × 10 ml vial);
        glucagon 1 mg (2 vials);
        dextrose 50% in 50 ml (2 vials).

Bibliography

Maloney ME. *The Dermatologic Surgical Suite. Design and Materials*. New York: Churchill Livingstone, 1991.

Drake LA, Ceilly RI, Cornelison RL *et al*. Guidelines of care for office surgical facilities. Part 2. Self-assessment checklist. *J Am Acad Dermatol* 1995; 33: 265–70.

2 Sterilisation and control of infection

2.1 Procurement of sterile supplies

When surgery is practised in the hospital environment, the necessary sterile equipment can be readily obtained from the hospital central sterile supply department. It is useful to have packs made up containing those instruments that are most commonly used in dermatological surgery. Surgeons operating in general practice or in private practice may be able to obtain packs of sterile instruments from the local hospital central sterilising unit. If this is not possible, then the practitioner will have to autoclave his or her own instruments; boiling or immersion of instruments in antiseptic solutions is not adequate to ensure destruction of organisms, spores and vegetative pathogens.

2.2 Autoclaving procedures

Most autoclaves work on the principle of a pressure cooker, and use high-pressure steam to destroy micro-organisms. Other forms of autoclave, which use dry heat or gas sterilisation, are not usually available to the office practitioner. The Little Sister® series of autoclaves have a chamber size roomy enough for sterilising prepackaged sets of instruments, whereas with the smaller machines, instruments may have to be autoclaved individually immediately prior to use, or alternatively sealed in small paper pouches which maintain their sterility. The duration of the autoclave sterilising cycle varies, but for a typical machine running at a pressure of 2 atmospheres and a steam temperature of 121°C, 15 min is adequate for sterilisation. However, to this must be added 15 min for initial heating, and a further 5–15 min for cooling down, so that the total cycle lasts 35–45 min. Most surgical materials can be autoclaved in this way, including metal, cloth, paper, glassware and heat-resistant plastic. One disadvantage of this form of autoclaving is the dulling of cutting surfaces, for example of scissors, which is a consequence of repeated sterilisation.

Steam autoclaves should be run using distilled water, and require regular maintenance by the manufacturer in order to guarantee sterility of instruments. Of particular importance is the renewal of rubber seals around the loading port of the instrument. For many of the smaller autoclaves it is usually wise to include paper heat-sensitive strips, which indicate that sterilisation is complete.

Preparation of instruments for autoclaving

It is essential to remove all foreign matter and organic debris from instruments prior to autoclaving, as micro-organisms may otherwise be protected from the sterilisation process. Instruments should be soaked in an antiseptic solution such as Toticide® for 15 min to ensure elimination of the human immunodeficiency virus (HIV), and adherent debris should subsequently be removed using a scrubbing brush. Disinfectants should not be mixed with detergents for the purpose of washing instruments, unless it is known that the detergent does not inactivate the disinfectant and is compatible with it.

At no time should the hinge of surgical instruments be lubricated, since the lubricating compound may bake during autoclaving, resulting in stiffness of the mechanism. Instruments should be regularly inspected to make sure that scissors do not have nicks in the cutting surface which may damage tissue, and that the tips of forceps and artery forceps meet properly. Defective instruments should be discarded or returned to the manufacturer for repair.

2.3 Skin and surface disinfection

Chemical antiseptics

The common antiseptics used for skin cleansing include aqueous chlorhexidine gluconate, povidone iodine and alcohol; of these, chlorhexidine is probably the most widely used.

Chlorhexidine

Chlorhexidine 4% aqueous solution is effective against a wide variety of bacteria, moulds, yeasts and viruses. Furthermore, chlorhexidine binds to proteins in the stratum corneum, leaving a persistent residue of antiseptic which is not subject to removal with alcohol. Chlorhexidine has a good safety record, with a very low incidence of irritation, allergy or photosensitivity, and does not appear to be absorbed through the skin to any significant degree. Chlorhexidine solutions come in both aqueous (Hibiscrub®, Hydrex®, Surgiscrub®) and alcoholic forms (Hibisol®), and it is essential to avoid the use of the alcoholic solutions when using cautery or electrosurgical devices. Alcoholic solutions also cause irritation to eyes and mucous membranes and even when only inhaled can cause headache and drowsiness, making them suitable for use only in well-ventilated spaces, free from electrosurgical devices or other ignition sources. Chlorhexidine is relatively non-toxic, but should not be allowed to come in contact with eyes, middle ear or brain tissues.

Povidone iodine

Povidone iodine 10% aqueous solution (Betadine® antiseptic solution) is the most frequently used iodine compound; it too is effective against a wide range of bacteria, viruses and spores. It is available as a surgical scrub (Betadine® surgical scrub) and as an alcoholic solution (Betadine® alcoholic solution). A potential problem with povidone iodine is that disinfection is achieved only after 15 min of moist contact with the skin, and povidone iodine may not remain stable for long periods. Other potential difficulties with povidone iodine include a relatively high incidence of skin reactions, and tissue irritation when the antiseptic is applied to broken skin. Povidine iodine can be inactivated by organic matter, and has the disadvantage that it may stain or corrode metal equipment.

Alcohol solutions

While 70% ethanol in aqueous solution can destroy 90% of bacteria in 2 min of continuous application, the usual single wipe with alcohol probably reduces skin flora by no more than 75%. Alcohol has the other disadvantage of precipitating protein, thereby causing damage in open wounds; moreover, alcoholic solutions may ignite in the presence of cautery or the electrical spark from a hyfrecator, with consequent risk of burns. Alcoholic solutions are useful, however, in disinfecting physically clean surfaces or equipment.

Chlorine-based disinfectants

Usually used in the form of a hypochloride solution (Milton®, Demestos®, Chloros®), powder (Septonite®, Diversol BX®) or granules (Prescept®, Titan®), chlorine-based disinfectants are particularly useful for dealing with contaminated spills on hard surfaces, but have the disadvantages of being corrosive to rubber, plastics and metals, and of bleaching fabrics. They must be made up to the recommended concentration just before use and are rapidly inactivated by organic matter.

Phenolic disinfectants

Used in concentrations of 1–2%, phenolic disinfectants (Stericol®, Hycolin®) are useful in the cleaning of surfaces or dealing with contaminated spillage. They are very irritant and must not come in contact with skin, or be used on equipment likely to come in contact with skin or mucous membranes. They are adsorbed by rubber and plastics, to which they can cause long-term damage.

Skin disinfection

The skin has a resident flora of bacteria, the nature of which depends on the site of the skin involved. While most of the resident flora inhabits the skin surface, some 20% of organisms reside in deeper layers of the skin, principally in the pilosebaceous units. It is impossible to remove all these organisms completely, but topical antiseptics can markedly reduce the number of pathogenic organisms on the skin surface. Clearly, the two areas where reduction in skin flora is necessary or desirable are on the surgeon's hands and on the patient's skin surrounding the field of surgery. Although use of sterile gloves is a cornerstone of aseptic technique, disinfection of the surgeon's hands is still required because bacteria multiply rapidly under gloves, and therefore glove puncture, which is a frequent occurrence, can lead to considerable wound contamination. It is generally held that hand washing with an aqueous detergent solution of chlorhexidine (Hibiscrub®, Hydrex®, Surgiscrub®) under a stream of running water provides sufficient disinfection. It may also be useful to consider using relatively small single-use sachets (e.g. Tisept®, Savlodil®) or plastic ampoules (e.g. Steripod®), each containing both chlorhexidine and cetrimide, as these are convenient for providing a ready supply of sterile solution when undertaking frequent but relatively small skin procedures. All antiseptic solutions must be used at their appropriate concentrations and must not be used following the expiry date stated on the container.

Patient preparation

Hair removal can often be avoided during cutaneous surgery, but when felt to be necessary it is probably best carried out prior to the operation. Shaving of hair can produce microtrauma to the skin, and thus increase the risk of bacterial infection. Clipping of hair avoids this complication and is therefore preferable; where hair is cosmetically important, such as the eyebrows, plucking, which encourages the hair follicle to go into the anagen or growth phase and therefore regrow quickly, is to be recommended.

Operating environment and surgical scrubbing

There is much controversy concerning many of the routine practices used in theatre environments, many of which are carried on through a sense of ritual rather than that based on sound microbiological study.

While it may be possible to achieve sterility in the theatre environment, neither the patient nor the staff can be sterilised. The majority of the bacteria in the air or on surfaces are derived from the skin, which is shed continuously, aided by movement and rubbing of clothes, as well as soon after bathing. People are thus the main source of bacteria in a theatre setting, and their number and movement in theatre should be limited. There is little evidence that wearing special theatre clothing offers significant microbiological advantage, and may, after a few hours, shed as much bacteria as normal clothing; they do, however, prevent contamination of normal clothes with blood and body fluids, and for this reason should be worn. It has long been traditional to wear face masks while in a theatre setting. The wearing of masks to protect the patient from infection shed from the surgeon's airway has not been proven to be effective, and studies have shown that bacterial counts in operating rooms are similar, and wound infection rates may even be less when masks are not worn. However, wearing of a mask may prevent contamination of the operator's mouth or nasal passages with blood or other fluids which may become airborne during a more extensive surgical intervention.

Surgical scrubbing is used to decrease the resident flora of the surgeon's or nurse's hands. All jewellery should be removed, and hands washed in an antiseptic solution from an elbow or foot-operated pump. The antiseptic can be applied as a lather for 1 min, and at the commencement of a list, nails may be gently scrubbed using a sterile brush to remove dirt that is ingrained or trapped under the nails. Vigorous 'scrubbing up' should be avoided as it may traumatise skin and probably does not improve on hand washing in antiseptic. A disposable sterile combined brush and sponge is available, which comes either with or without impregnated chlorhexidine gluconate (E-Z scrub®). After washing in running water, the hands should be washed for a further 2 min, before drying using sterile paper towels and putting on sterile gloves.

2.4 Surgical drapes

The use of sterile drapes is essential to ensure a sterile field of work (see Section 1.6).

2.5 Antibiotics and routine skin surgery

Antibiotics are generally not required for minor operative procedures, and sterile technique during surgery is preferable to the use of antibiotics afterwards. Oral antibiotics such as erythromycin, amoxycillin or cephalexin may, however, be advisable during prolonged operative procedures, such as micrographic (Mohs') surgery or reconstructive surgery, where the risk of infection may be greater, and the consequences more disastrous should it occur. They may also be indicated for patients undergoing delayed closure of a wound or following evacuation of a haematoma. In addition, prophylaxis may sometimes be considered useful for incisional surgery involving the oronasal mucosa, perineal area or axillae, where skin is usually contaminated with high numbers of bacteria. Prophylaxis should commence 1 h prior to surgery to ensure that adequate tissue levels of the antibiotic are achieved. For most skin surgery, antibiotics need only be given for 24 h.

Some simple measures can be taken to decrease the possibility of perioperative infection generally. These include showering on the day before surgery with an antiseptic soap, applying topical antibiotics (chosen on the basis of results of bacterial culture swabs), and deferring elective surgery in patients with known infections.

If infection does occur, then *Staphylococcus aureus* or *Streptococcus pyogenes* are the usual culprits and erythromycin, amoxycillin or cephalexin may be used in doses of 250–500 mg four times daily for 10 days. The choice of antibiotic agent should be made from the results of bacteriological cultures of infected wound material or swabs, where this is possible. Infection of cartilage or bone is usually more serious and may require the addition of 500 mg fusidic acid four times daily for 10 days if the infection is deemed to be severe.

2.6 Prophylaxis for bacterial endocarditis

It is important to remember that patients with certain abnormalities of the cardiovascular system, including those with prosthetic heart valves, patent ductus arteriosus and mitral or aortic valve disease, are at high risk of developing endocarditis, and may require preoperative antibiotic therapy. Patients with other heart abnormalities, such as mitral valve prolapse without valvular regurgitation, tricuspid and pulmonary valve disease, or those who have a cardiac pacemaker, are at low risk of developing endocarditis and do not require antibiotic prophylaxis. Unfortunately, no definitive guidelines exist regarding antibiotic prophylaxis during skin surgery, and the following recommendations are based on a review of the current literature. It must, therefore, be emphasised that if any uncertainty exists regarding a patient, it is recommended that the surgeon should liaise with the patient's cardiologist before elective surgery is undertaken.

Recent studies have shown that bacteraemia occurring during skin surgery on clinically non-infected, non-ulcerated skin lesions is low, being less than 1%, and in such cases prophylactic antibiotics do not seem to be warranted. Thus, even in patients with a high risk of developing endocarditis, perioperative antibiotics are probably not required for minor surgery (punch biopsy, curettage and cautery, shave excision, cryosurgery, laser surgery or simple incisions lasting less than 20 min) on non-infected, intact skin lesions. However, surgery or manipulation of clinically infected or ulcerated skin lesions is associated with a high incidence of bacteraemia with organisms which may result in endocarditis. Thus, perioperative antibiotics are considered advisable in patients who are at high risk of developing endocarditis, or are undergoing operations on infected or ulcerated skin lesions, prolonged surgery, surgery in areas of high bacterial contamination (oronasal mucosa, perineum or axillae), or where wound defects are being left to heal by secondary intention.

Controversy also exists regarding antibiotic regimens suitable for patients with a high risk of developing endocarditis. The following regimens seem most appropriate. For each antibiotic regimen the preoperative dose of antibiotic should be administered 1 h before surgery with a further dose 6 h postoperatively. The optimum agent effective against organisms (including methicillin-resistant *Staphylococcus aureus*) encountered in infected skin lesions is vancomycin (500 mg preoperatively and 250 mg postoperatively). The disadvantages of vancomycin are that is must be given by slow intravenous infusion over 1 h, is expensive and may cause hypotension or skin rashes. Less effective regimens are cephalexin or flucloxacillin (500 mg administered preoperatively and postoperatively) or intravenous clindamycin (500 mg preoperatively and 150 mg postoperatively). Where surgery involves the oronasal mucosa, then 3 g oral amoxycillin administered preoperatively and 1.5 g postoperatively should suffice; in patients who are allergic to penicillin, erythromycin (1 g preoperatively and 500 g postoperatively) is a suitable alternative.

2.7 Prophylaxis for prostheses

As is the case for bacterial endocarditis, there are no specific recommendations regarding antibiotic prophylaxis in patients with artificial prostheses who are undergoing elective skin surgery. However, the current literature provides a number of guidelines, but if there is any uncertainty regarding a patient, it is recommended that the surgeon should liaise with the subspecialist involved in the patient's care, before elective surgery is undertaken.

Prophylactic antibiotics are usually necessary when undertaking surgery on patients with infected or ulcerated skin lesions who are undergoing haemodialysis with arteriovenous shunts. Similarly, antibiotics are recommended for patients who have orthopaedic prostheses or ventriculoatrial and peritoneal cerebrospinal fluid shunts, if infection or ulceration is present at the site of skin surgery. Patients with synthetic arterial grafts probably only warrant antibiotic prophylaxis during the first month after implantation (before the graft becomes endothelialised) and patients with breast implants or genitourinary prostheses (for example, penile catheters) seem to be at sufficiently low risk that perioperative antibiotics are not required.

Where antibiotics are required, the same regimens should be used as for the prophylaxis of bacterial endocarditis (see Section 2.6).

2.8 Protection for surgical personnel and laboratory staff

Over recent years, increasing attention has been paid to the potential risk of infection from hepatitis B and C virus or HIV to surgical personnel as a result of minor surgery. Infection of the surgeon can occur through blood contamination of broken skin, splashes on to the conjunctiva or oral mucosa or through needle-stick injury; laboratory staff are also at risk during handling of tissue. The viruses remain viable for some time following contamination of surfaces; HIV is viable for some 3 days in dried blood, whereas hepatitis B remains viable for 7 days. The risk of transmission of hepatitis B, hepatitis C and HIV after a sharps injury (needle-stick injury transfers approximately 1.4 µl blood) is probably of the order of 20%, 4% and 0.4%, respectively. It is essential that gloves be worn during every operative procedure. Some suggest the use of double gloving, which reduces the risk of contamination of the hands with blood and also probably reduces the number of needle-stick injuries; in addition, if perforation of both the inner and outer glove does occur, the perforation sites rarely match, thus providing protection from physical contact of the wound with blood. The wearing of goggles or visors may prevent conjunctival contamination with splashes of blood where a known risk of infection exists. Wounds or broken skin should be covered with a waterproof dressing, should be regularly washed between patients, and protective clothing should be worn when splashes with body fluids seem likely. All staff must be vigilant in the disposal of sharps into suitable containers, should avoid resheathing needles, should not fill sharps containers to more than three-quarters and should label specimens from patients who are infected, or potentially infected, with the viruses with biohazard labels. In the case of a patient known to be infected, all contaminated instruments and drapes should be placed in sealed plastic boxes marked with biohazard labelling before their return to the central sterile supply department. Contaminated spills must be dealt with by personnel wearing gloves and an apron, by wiping the surface using paper towels soaked in a hypochlorite-type disinfectant, which should then be disposed of in a plastic bag marked for use with clinical waste.

Perhaps the greatest risk to the surgeon is still that of hepatitis B infection. Therefore, all who are at occupational risk should be screened for immunity to the hepatitis B e antigen; personnel who are positive for this, or who refuse to take the test, must be deployed in a low-risk capacity. If a surgeon is found to be positive to hepatitis B e, the test should be repeated and confirmed on a further serum sample, perhaps best carried out at a different virology centre. It is now considered indefensible for a surgeon to perform 'invasive surgery' when hepatitis B e or HIV positive, although skin surgery may not necessarily fall into the category of 'invasive surgery'. Non-immune subjects should undergo vaccination with the now very safe, genetically engineered vaccine Engerix®. Arthritis, reactive arthritis and a Reiter's-type syndrome have recently been recorded only rarely with such vaccines. Seroconversion is of the order of 96%, and should be confirmed following the vaccination programme. A titre of hepatitis B surface antibody greater than 100 mIU/ml is regarded as indicating immunity; subjects achieving a titre of 50–100 mIU/ml are recommended to have a booster dose after 1 year, and those failing to respond can be given further doses, with some individuals requiring up to nine doses to achieve immunity.

Management of sharps injury

In the event of a needle-stick or similar injury, the wound should be encouraged to bleed and rinsed under running water. The wound should not be sucked or scrubbed, but may be washed in soap and water and dried. The Occupational Health Department should be contacted for advice and the hospital's infection control policy followed. Blood for hepatitis B and HIV testing can only be taken from the patient with informed consent. Serum hepatitis B immunoglobulin therapy (0.06 ml/kg body weight) should be offered following perioperative injury to an individual known to have no antibodies to the hepatitis B virus, and should be followed up 7 days later with the first dose of hepatitis B vaccine. Although of unproven benefit, it has been suggested that zidovudine (AZT) be offered to surgeons who suffer an injury or who are splashed with blood during surgery on a patient known to be HIV positive; 1 g of oral zidovudine may be taken within 2 h of the contamination, followed by a course of the drug at a dose of 250 mg four times a day for 28 days. It may be considered prudent to have 'starter packs' containing 1 g of zidovudine in theatre, so that a first dose may be taken quickly.

2.9 Surgical gloves

Gloves must provide an effective two-way barrier between the patient and the health care professional. Sterile gloves must be worn during aseptic procedures when infection transfer to the patient from the operator or environment is possible: non-sterile gloves may be used where primarily there is an infection risk to the operator and asepsis is not necessary. Latex gloves remain the most cost-effective and safest barrier for protecting both the patient and surgeon from infection, and must pass rigorous standards regarding physical thickness, strength and ability to withstand pressure and pass a water-tight leak test. There are several synthetic materials that have been used to substitute for latex in the manufacturing of surgical-type gloves, but in general these have not been found to be as effective in their barrier function when exposed to large amounts of blood and body fluids. Studies have shown that gloves that have been worn for long periods of time, especially more than 3 h, have a higher number of punctures than gloves worn for short periods.

Latex allergy

There has been an increasing awareness of latex allergy among health care professionals recently, with studies showing a 2.9–16% sensitivity to latex protein. Ideally, all hospital personnel should use hypoallergenic powder-free gloves which should have antigenic latex protein concentrations of less than 14 μg/g. Symptoms of latex protein allergy include contact urticaria, angioneurotic oedema, pruritus, urticaria, rhinitis, conjunctivitis, asthma and life-threatening anaphylaxis. Studies have shown that glove powder with corn starch used as a donning agent can cause an aerosoling of latex protein in the operating theatre such that the latex becomes an inhaled aeroallergen.

In addition to health care workers, patients with spina bifida, who have undergone multiple surgical procedures and patients with atopy may all be sensitised from latex contact in high exposure.

Diagnosis and precautions for latex allergy

In a person suspected of having latex allergy, skin prick testing should be used. Protein should be eluted from the gloves by cutting 1 g of glove into small pieces and soaking them at room temperature in 5 ml of physiological saline for 15 min. After this, the solution may be used for performing prick testing on the forearm with saline as a negative control and histamine as a positive control. Blood serum may also be submitted for radioallergosorbent tests (RASTs) for latex: this method has an 80% sensitivity and 100% specificity in non-atopic individuals. If necessary, a challenge test can be carried out where the person wears a finger of the latex glove on one hand while using a finger of polyvinyl chloride (PVC) glove on the other as a negative control. Skin can be examined after 15 min to see if any changes have occurred. The challenge test can be used when the skin prick test is not in accordance with the clinical history or in those with weakly positive skin prick tests or RASTs, as well as in those who are thought to be allergic to the gloves but remain negative on testing. The use of a challenge test should only be carried out with adequate equipment necessary to treat anaphylaxis should this occur.

When operating on someone who is allergic to latex it is important to avoid contact with all latex products during the perioperative period, including examination gloves, latex tubing, rubber ports used to administer intravenous drugs, rubber stoppers on many injection vials and the use of non-latex catheter equipment.

For theatre personnel who are allergic to latex protein, suitable surgical gloves include Derma-Prene®, Medigrip® (Ansell), Biogel® (Regent) and Allegard® (a new synthetic surgical glove) (Johnson & Johnson).

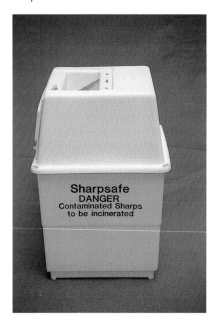

Fig. 2.1 Small plastic sharps disposal box.

2.10 Sharps and waste disposal

Sharps

Sharp instruments, including all needles, scalpel blades, syringes or broken glassware must be disposed of safely by the person who uses them; it is not defensible to delegate this to others. Needles should not be detached from syringes or resheathed before disposal. If a sharp is lost, the person responsible for its use must inform all other members of staff, including cleaners, etc., so that they can take due care until it is found.

Sharps should be disposed of into a sharps box, conforming to British Standard 3720 (Fig. 2.1), or similar standard in other countries. The sharps box should be closed when 75% full, and then sent for incineration.

Clinical waste

All tissue, soiled dressings, swabs and drapes must be disposed of by personnel wearing gloves into designated clinical waste bags; in the United Kingdom these are yellow in colour (British Standard 309), of minimum gauge 100 (25 µm), marked 'clinical waste' and of maximum nominal capacity 0.1 m³. Bags must be closed when they are 75% full and handled only by those wearing heavy duty protective clothing. Purpose-made plastic ties should be used for sealing the bags, which must then be sent for incineration.

Bibliography

Benedetto AV, Griffin TD, Beneddeto EA, Humeniuk HM. Dermabrasion: therapy and prophylaxis of the photoaged face. *J Am Acad Dermatol* 1992; 27: 439–47.

Buback ME, Reid CE, Fansway FA *et al.* Allergic reactions to latex among health care workers. *Mayo Clin Proc* 1992; 67: 1075–9.

Carmichael AJ, Flanagan PG, Holt PJA *et al.* The occurrence of bacteraemia with skin surgery. *Br J Dermatol* 1996;134: 120–2.

Delamothe T. Hepatitis B and exposure prone procedures. *Br Med J* (Editorial) 1994; 309: 73–4.

Dias M, Conchon I, Cortes M, Pereira F, Alonso R. Anaphylactic interoperative reaction to latex. *Contact Dermatitis* 1995; 32: 303–6.

Gazzard GB, Wastell C. HIV and surgeons. *Br Med J* 1990; 301: 1003–4.

Hanque KN, Chagla AH. Do gowns prevent infection in neonatal intensive care units? *J Hosp Infect* 1989; 14: 159–62.

Hassan W, Oldham R. Reiter's syndrome and reactive arthritis in health care workers after vaccination. *Br Med J* 1994; 309: 94.

Joint Working Party of the Hospital Infection Society and Surgical Infection Study Group. Risk to surgeons and patients from HIV and hepatitis: guidelines on precautions and management of exposure to blood or body fluids. *Br Med J* 1992; 305: 1337–43.

Kiene K, Hsu B, Rowe D. Hepatitis, HIV, and the dermatologist: a risk review. *J Am Acad Dermatol* 1994; 30: 108–15.

Korniewicz DM, Laughon B, Cyr H, Lytle CD, Larson E. Leakage of virus through used vial and latex examination gloves. *J Clin Microbiol* 1990; 28: 787–8.

Meers PD, Yeo GA. Shedding of bacteria and skin squames after hand washing. *J Hyg Camb* 1978; 81: 81–6.

Myers SA, Prose NS, Bartlett JA. Progress in the understanding of HIV infection: an overview. *J Am Acad Dermatol* 1993; 29: 1–21.

Ojajarvi J, Makela P, Rantasalo I. Failure of hand disinfection with frequent handwashing: a need for prolonged field studies. *J Hyg Camb* 1997; 79: 107–19.

Orr NWM. Is a mask necessary in the operating theatre? *Ann Roy Coll Surg Engl* 1981; 63: 390–1.

Poole CJM., Miller S, Fillingham G. Immunity to hepatitis B among health care workers performing exposure prone procedures. *Br Med J* 1994; 309: 94–5.

Reybrouck G. Handwashing and hand disinfection. *J Hosp Infect* 1986; 8: 5–23.

Ritter MA, Eitzen H, French ML, Hart JB. The operating room environment as affected by people and the surgical face mask. *Clin Orthop* 1975; 111: 147–50.

Sabetta JB, Zitelli JA. The incidence of bacteraemia during skin surgery. *Arch Dermatol* 1987; 123: 213–15.

Sebben JE. Sterilization and care of surgical instruments and supplies. *J Am Acad Dermatol* 1984; 11: 381–92.

Sebben JE. Sterile technique and the prevention of wound infection in office surgery (Part I). *J Dermatol Surg Oncol* 1988; 14: 1364–71.

Sebben JE. Sterile technique in dermatologic surgery: what is enough? *J Dermatol Surg Oncol* 1988; 14: 487–9.

Sebben JE. Sterile technique and the prevention of wound infection in office surgery (Part II). *J Dermatol Surg Oncol* 1989; 15: 38–48.

Sebben JE, Davis CA. Surgical antiseptics. *J Am Acad Dermatol* 1983; 9: 759–65.

Simmons BP. Guidelines for hospital environmental control. *Infect Control Hosp Epidemiol* 1982; 2: 131–7.

Turner MJ, Crowley P, MacDonald D. The unmasking of delivery room routine. *J Obs Gynaecol* 1984; 4: 188–90.

Wagner RF, Grande DJ, Feingold DS. Antibiotic prophylaxis against bacterial endocarditis in patients undergoing dermatological surgery. *Arch Dermatol* 1986; 122: 799–801.

Yunginger JW, Jones RT, Fransway AF, Kelso JM, Warner MA, Hunt LW. Extractable latex allergens and proteins in disposable medical gloves and other rubber products. *J Allergy Clin Immunol* 1994; 93: 836–8.

3 Anatomy for skin surgery

A fairly detailed knowledge of anatomy is necessary for a skin surgeon, as it allows work to be carried out safely, enables planning of regional anaesthesia and ensures that there is no residual functional impairment of important structures, such as eyelids, lips or underlying nerves. For most skin surgery, there are only a relatively small number of important structures that must be avoided or handled with care. The main emphasis of this chapter will be on the head and neck, in view of the relative frequency of skin surgery to these areas. The nomenclature of subregions of the head and neck is illustrated in Figs 3.1 and 3.2.

3.1 Surface anatomy

Certain important landmarks on the head and neck may be readily delineated in relation to fixed bony structures. At the midpoint of the supraorbital margin, in line with the pupil, lies the supraorbital foramen, which is easily palpable; from this orifice, the supraorbital nerve emerges to run anteriorly onto the forehead. Approximately 1 cm inferior to the infraorbital margin, in the line of the pupil, lies the infraorbital foramen, which transmits the infraorbital vessels and nerves; it is usually readily palpable in the central cheek region. The mental foramen, from which issues the mental nerve, is situated at the midpoint of the mandible, in the mid-pupillary line just below the first pre-molar tooth. Each of these landmarks lies some 2.5 cm from the midline; their relationship to the surface anatomy and underlying bones is shown in Fig. 3.3.

The zygomatic arch is a prominent bony structure which runs from the malar eminence to the external auditory meatus. It is the attachment for the masseter muscle, itself an important landmark in the facial area, since it enables delineation of important nerves and vessels as they cross the zygomatic arch superficially before entering the temple region. The masseter muscle can be clearly felt beneath the zygomatic arch coursing downwards towards the mandible; its anterior border becomes obvious when the teeth are clenched. This muscle is important as the parotid gland lies on its posterior half, and the parotid duct crosses the masseter muscle at the tragolabial line, before curving medially around its anterior border to pierce the buccinator muscle, and enter the mouth at the level of the second upper molar tooth. The parotid duct is vulnerable to injury at this site and it is obviously important to be aware of these structures while carrying out deep surgery in this area (Fig. 3.4). Another important structure in this region is the superficial temporal artery. The artery can be palpated as it crosses the zygomatic arch just anterior to the external ear. It divides in this region into its anterior branch, which courses across the forehead, and its parietal branch, which continues upwards onto the scalp (Fig. 3.4).

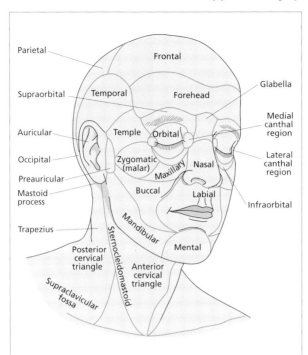

Fig. 3.1 Surface compartments of the head and neck.

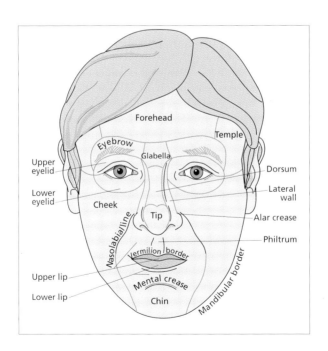

Fig. 3.2 Surface compartments of the face.

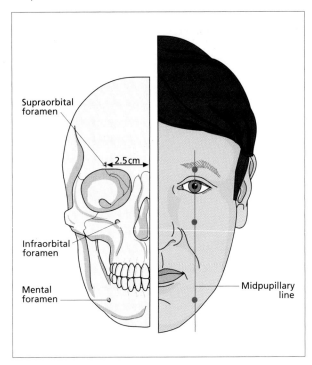

Fig. 3.3 Important bony landmarks in relation to nerve foramina.

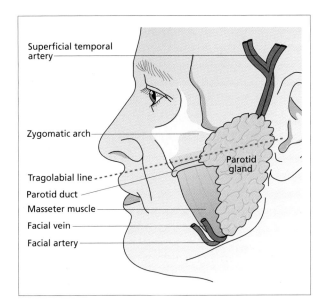

Fig. 3.4 Structures of importance in the region of the zygomatic arch.

3.2 The facial nerve

The facial nerve enters the face by passing through the deep substance of the parotid gland, where it divides into its five terminal branches, which exit the gland on their way to supply the muscles of facial expression, as well as to provide sensory innervation for the anterior two-thirds of the

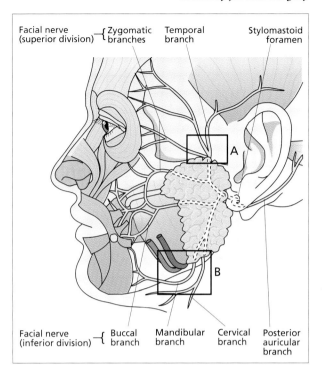

Facial nerve (superior division) — Zygomatic branches   Temporal branch   Stylomastoid foramen

A

B

Facial nerve (inferior division) — Buccal branch   Mandibular branch   Cervical branch   Posterior auricular branch

Fig. 3.5 Branches of the facial nerve with danger zones shown in areas A and B.

tongue, the external auditory meatus, soft palate and pharynx. The zygomatic, buccal and cervical branches run deep after their exit from the parotid gland, being covered by the masseter muscle and by fascia. However, both the temporal branch and the mandibular branches of the facial nerve lie more superficially, and are easily damaged during skin surgery, making knowledge of their anatomy vital.

The temporal branch of the facial nerve crosses the zygomatic arch before traversing anteriorly and diagonally across the temple just below the superficial temporalis fascia. This branch of the facial nerve is most at risk of being cut as it crosses the middle of the zygomatic arch, especially in patients who are thin and cachectic (danger zone A highlighted in Fig. 3.5). Injury to this nerve results in ipsilateral inability to wrinkle the forehead and raise the eyebrow.

The marginal mandibular branch of the facial nerve exits the parotid gland at the angle of the jaw where it lies relatively unprotected on the external surface of the masseter muscle, covered only by skin, subcutaneous tissue and fascia. As it courses anteriorly, it is covered by the platysma muscle, but it is at risk of damage at the angle of the jaw (danger zone B highlighted in Fig. 3.5), with resultant drooping of the corner of the mouth.

3.3 Blood vessels of the face

Most of the blood supply to the head and neck is delivered by branches of the external carotid artery (Fig. 3.6). The terminal branch of the external

33

carotid artery, the superficial temporal artery, has already been described as it passes over the zygomatic arch anterior to the external ear to divide into its two terminal branches. The other major artery in the area is the facial artery, which arises from the anterior border of the external carotid artery, from which it courses anteriorly, and upwards over the mandible, to enter the face immediately anterior to the masseter muscle, where it can be easily palpated (Fig. 3.7a). The facial artery then crosses the face diagonally to the angle of the mouth and upwards and onwards to the inner canthus of the eye (Fig. 3.7a,b). From the anterior surface of the facial artery arise the inferior and superior labial arteries. After the superior labial artery has branched off, the facial artery becomes the angular artery, which continues on across the medial canthal area to terminate at the root of the nose. The

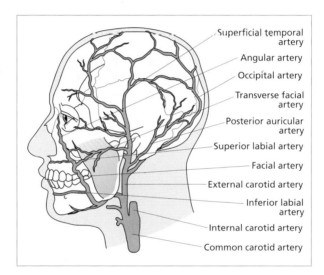

Fig. 3.6 The arterial supply of head and neck.

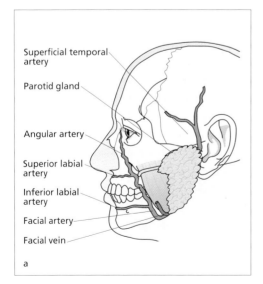

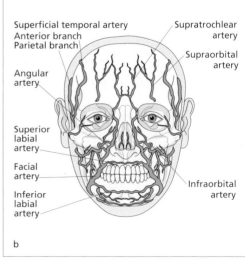

Fig. 3.7 a, b. Arterial supply of the face.

two labial arteries course through the centre of the lips on the mucosal side, and lie on the inner surface of the muscle layer some 0.5 cm below the ver- milion border. It is important to identify and ligate these during wedge resection of the lip.

Other branches of the external carotid artery are perhaps less important for the dermatological surgeon, but one that deserves mention is the occip- ital artery. This leaves the posterior aspect of the carotid artery at the same level as the facial artery, exits from the posterior border of the sternocleido- mastoid muscle, and runs posteriorly and superiorly onto the occipital scalp.

The venous drainage of the face by and large follows the path of the arterial system. Unlike the veins on the trunk and extremities, the facial veins do not have valves. This is important, since the facial vein communi- cates with the ophthalmic vein, resulting in direct connection between the external veins of the face and the cavernous sinus. This in turn raises the possibility of infection tracking through the connection, leading to the seri- ous complication of cavernous sinus thrombosis.

3.4 Lymphatic drainage of the head and neck

The lymphatic system of the head and neck can be conveniently thought of as being divided into horizontally and vertically arranged groups of lymph nodes (Fig. 3.8). The horizontal group of lymph nodes encircles the junction of the head and the neck, and includes the submental and submandibular glands lying beneath the mandible, the superficial parotid

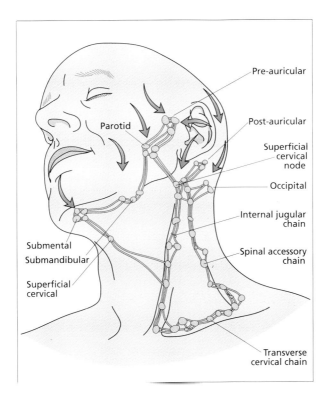

Fig. 3.8 Lymphatic drainage of the head and neck.

(pre-auricular) lying anterior to the ear and the mastoid and occipital nodes lying in the posterior triangle of the neck just below the hairline. These lymph nodes, which drain the superficial tissues of the head and neck, in turn drain into the deep cervical nodes, which extend down from the base of the skull to the root of the neck, along the line of the internal jugular vein and external carotid artery. From here, the lymph passes via the jugular trunk to the thoracic duct or the right lymphatic duct.

Familiarity with regional fields of lymphatic drainage of the skin in the clinical assessment of cutaneous malignancies (e.g. squamous cell carcinoma or melanoma) on the head and neck area is clearly important, so that the appropriate lymph nodes can be carefully checked. It is also essential for proper planning of lymph node dissection or radiotherapy, and for the instruction of patients on massage to relieve lymphoedema. The submental nodes anteriorly drain the middle two-thirds of the lower lip, as well as the anterior floor of the mouth and anterior one-third of the tongue. The submandibular nodes drain most of the lower face, cheek and nose, while the anterior scalp, posterior cheek and anterior ear drain to the pre-auricular and parotid nodes. The middle one-third of the scalp drains to the posterior auricular nodes, while the posterior part of the scalp drains to the occipital nodes (Fig. 3.8). After these primary lymph nodes are affected by tumour, further progression into the deep cervical nodes is the rule.

To adequately detect submental lymph nodes when they are small, bimanual palpation must be used which involves placing one finger under the tongue, behind the lower teeth or uvular rim and palpating the opposite finger placed externally in the submental area.

3.5 Regional head and neck anatomy

The scalp

The skin of the scalp extends from the supra-orbital ridge anteriorly to the superior nuchal line of the occipital bone, and is unremarkable apart from its large number of hair follicles. Below the dermis lies a musculo-aponeurotic layer, consisting of muscle between two layers of fascia. The muscle layer is present anteriorly and posteriorly, but is absent over the greater part of the top of the skull; here, the two layers of fascia fuse to form the galea aponeurotica, beneath which lies only loose connective tissue above the periosteum of the scalp. The subgaleal space is important, as it is the usual level for undermining on the scalp. In addition, it constitutes a large area where subgaleal haematoma can form; infection in this area can progress through emissary veins to enter the intracranial venous sinuses.

The sensory supply of the scalp arises from a large number of nerves, which enter the region around the hairline, in the subcutaneous fat layer. Field block for the scalp can therefore be achieved by local infiltration of the subcutaneous compartment in a ring manner around the scalp, when extensive procedures are anticipated.

The blood supply to the scalp is rich, with an anastomotic network of vessels in the subcutaneous plane. This makes flaps on the scalp relatively easy to design, without fear of compromising their blood supply.

The external eye

The anterior surface of the eye is protected by its upper and lower lids. The main support structures of both upper and lower eyelids are the tarsal plates: crescent-shaped structures comprised of dense fibrous tissue which lie in the posterior third of each eyelid. The skin of the eyelids is thin, overlying loosely attached muscle. The lid margins at the junction between the skin and the mucous membrane of the conjunctiva (the so-called grey line) are some 2 mm wide. From these margins, the eyelashes emerge as two or three irregular rows; the sebaceous glands of Zeis open onto the lid margins. On the posterior aspect of the lid lie the Meibomian glands, which can be seen as yellow streaks on the inner surface of the lids; they may undergo cystic retention changes.

Full thickness excisions of lid margins, which should be orientated vertically, must include repair of the tarsal plate. The upper lid usually has much more redundant skin than the lower lid, making surgical intervention easier. The development of ectropion is a potential hazard with all surgery of the lower eyelid.

From the surgical point of view, most of the important structures lie medially with the lacrimal drainage system (Fig. 3.9). From puncta which lie on the conjunctival surface of the upper and lower eyelids, canaliculi

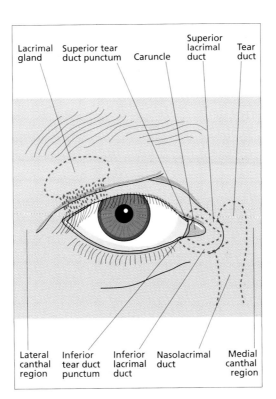

Fig. 3.9 Important anatomical structures in relation to the eye.

progress in a vertical direction for some 2 mm, before taking a 90° turn and travelling horizontally for some 8 mm, to end under the medial canthal tendon in the tear sac. Placing a probe in the canaliculi helps to define them during surgery in this area. From the tear sac, the nasolacrimal duct arises and travels inferiorly to open into the nose below the inferior turbinate.

The nose

The surface anatomy of the nose is illustrated in Fig. 3.10. The upper one-third of the nose is supported by firm, paired nasal bones, whereas the lower two-thirds has a cartilaginous support from the lateral and alar cartilages, and a single septal cartilage. Over the bony area the skin is loose and easily undermined, whereas on the lower two-thirds of the nose the skin is firmly bound down, making anaesthesia and undermining in this area difficult. Viewed from below, each nasal opening is bounded medially by the columella, laterally by the alar rim, and inferiorly and posteriorly by the nostril sill. The nose has a rich blood supply, much of it derived from the terminal branch of the facial artery, the angular artery. Thus, in general, the nose (especially the upper part) heals well, but the free edge of the nostril rim is prone to healing with notching and retraction. The cutaneous innervation of the nose is provided by several different nerves, although much of the side wall of the nose is innervated by branches of the infraorbital nerve (Fig. 3.11).

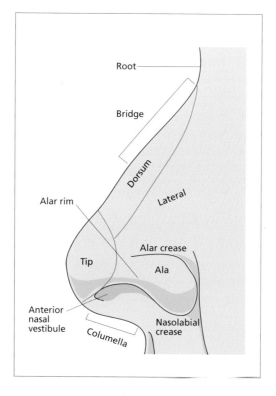

Fig. 3.10 The surface anatomy of the nose.

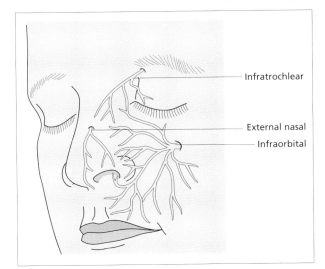

Fig. 3.11
Cutaneous
innervation of the
nose.

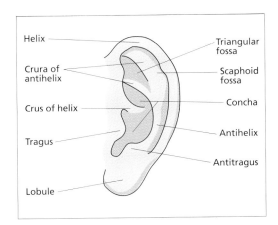

Fig. 3.12 Anatomical areas
of the external ear.

The ear

The anatomy of the external ear is shown in Fig. 3.12. The external ear has a rich blood supply; the anterior section being supplied from branches of the superficial temporal artery, and the posterior part via branches of the posterior auricular artery. The skin is tightly adherent to the underlying cartilage, especially anteriorly, making local anaesthesia in this area difficult. Because the ear is supplied by a number of different sensory nerves, it is necessary to inject local anaesthetic in a ring around the base of the ear in order to achieve a field block; for total anaesthesia, further anaesthetic should be injected subdermally anterior to the concha.

Posterior triangle of the neck

The posterior triangle of the neck is bounded anteriorly by the sternomastoid muscle, inferiorly by the clavicle and posteriorly by the trapezius muscle. The triangle is traversed by the spinal accessory nerve, which in this

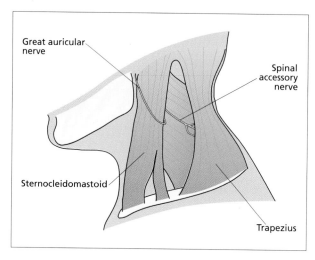

Great auricular nerve

Spinal accessory nerve

Sternocleidomastoid

Trapezius

Fig. 3.13 Posterior triangle of neck with spinal accessory and great auricular nerves.

region is covered only by skin and subcutaneous fascia. The nerve is thus in danger of division here (Fig. 3.13), especially in thin individuals, with resultant drooping of the shoulder or development of a frozen shoulder because of decreased muscle activity.

3.6 Limb anatomy

The upper limb

Dermatological surgery of the limbs is in general not particularly hazardous, as there are few vital structures that lie superficially and are thus at risk. It is, however, possible to expose and damage the lower branches of the brachial plexus when removing skin deeply in the axilla, as for hyperhidrosis, especially in thin patients. Such injury would result in anaesthesia of the ulnar border of the arm, and weakness and wasting of the smooth muscles of the hand. The ulnar nerve is at risk as it passes behind the medial epicondyle, where it can be readily felt against the bone, to enter the forearm. Damage to the nerve at this site causes paralysis of the fourth and fifth fingers with a claw deformity to the hand.

The lymphatics of both the dorsal and ventral surfaces of the forearm and of the hand drain to the supratrochlear lymph nodes just above the medial aspect of the elbow. These nodes in turn drain to the lateral axillary nodes. The lymphatics of the upper arm and shoulder region drain to the medial and posterior axillary lymph nodes.

The lower limb

The common peroneal nerve, which can be felt against the bone as it winds its way round the neck of the fibula, is at risk of damage during deep incisions through the subcutaneous fat in this area, resulting in a permanent foot drop. Damage may also follow tight plaster casts or bandages around the leg at this site. The majority of the plantar surface of the foot is innervated by the posterior tibial nerve, only small areas of the medial and later-

al surfaces of the foot are not supplied by this nerve. It arises in the sciatic nerve, and descends along the posterior calf to the ankle, where it passes between the Achilles tendon and the medial malleolus, immediately poste-rior to the posterior tibial artery and deep to the flexor retinaculum. At this site, it is possible to perform a nerve block to provide anaesthesia to the sole of the foot.

The lymphatic drainage of the lower limbs passes through a group of lymphatics arranged medially around the knee and onwards and upwards to the superficial inguinal nodes, which are arranged in a chain imme-diately below the inguinal ligament. The superficial inguinal nodes also receive drainage from the anterior abdominal wall below the umbilicus, the external genitalia and the lower anal canal and peri-anal region.

The digits

The anatomy of the nerve and blood supply to the fingers and toes is essentially the same. Both have two dorsal and two ventral nerves and corresponding digital arteries, which are in turn supplied by arterial arches. In the hand, these arterial arches are supplied by two arteries, namely the terminal branches of the radial and ulnar arteries, while in the foot the plantar arterial arches are formed as the terminal branches of the lateral and medial plantar arteries.

3.7 Relaxed skin tension lines

The relaxed skin tension lines (RSTLs) are related to the underlying musculature and joints. Often they are related to creases that develop in the skin, especially of the head and neck, as a result of the decreased elastic tissue tone, and lengthened collagenous fibrous septa, associated with the ageing process and solar damage to the skin. Perhaps the easiest way to become familiar with the orientation of RSTLs is to study the skin of elderly people. They usually lie perpendicular to the underlying muscle groups. For the best cosmetic results, an incisional scar should be placed along or within a RSTL; this will tend to conceal the scar, especially in the elderly patient where skin creases are well developed. When operating on a patient in which the RSTLs are not well developed, their direction can usually be ascertained by pinching the skin between the thumb and forefinger. If the pinching is parallel to the RSTLs, then fine parallel wrinkles will be seen, whereas if it is across the lines, a twisted S-shape line will result. Another method of ascertaining the RSTLs direction is to ask the patient to smile or frown. Alternatively, a lesion may be excised as a circular defect, and after the surrounding skin is undermined, the wound will often form an oval shape with the long axis in the direction of the RSTL.

Some general rules can be stated and are shown in Figs 3.14 and 3.15. For example, RSTLs tend to be transverse on the forehead, but vertical or oblique in the glabellar region (Fig. 3.14). On the upper nose they are hori-zontal, on the side walls they are oblique and on the bridge of the nose they become vertical. On the cheek these lines are often curvilinear, while on the lips they tend to radiate from the vermilion border. On the extremities,

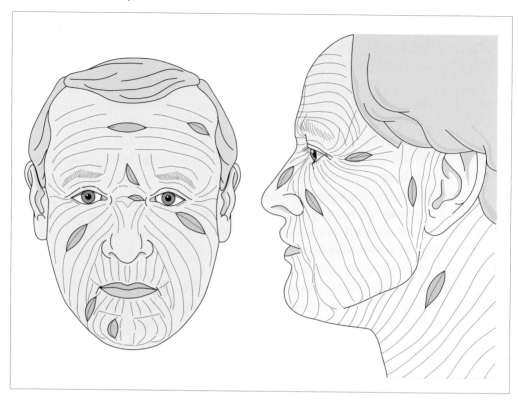

Fig. 3.14 Relaxed skin tension lines on facial areas.

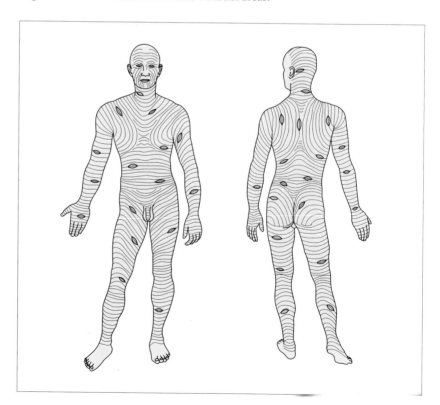

Fig. 3.15 Relaxed skin tension lines on the body and limbs.

the RSTLs are usually circumferential (Fig. 3.15). On the trunk it may be difficult to determine their direction; they tend to be vertical on the upper back and on the lateral chest wall, whereas around the central trunk they tend to be circumferential.

3.8 Cosmetic units

The face consists of a number of well-defined cosmetic regions or units, each with its own individual characteristics in terms of skin colour, elasticity, texture and thickness, sebaceous gland prominence and hairiness. The boundaries between these are usually well defined, and include the contour lines of the nasofacial sulcus, the philtral ridge, the nasolabial folds, the glabellar area and the temple. Scars should be sited where possible along such junctions, in order to conceal them. It is also preferable not to move skin from one cosmetic unit to another because of the difference in characteristics.

Bibliography

Bernstein G. Surface landmarks for the identification of key anatomic structures of the face and neck. *J Dermatol Surg Oncol* 1986; 12: 7.

Hosal IN, Onerci M, Kayas A, Turan E. Squamous cell carcinoma of the lower lip. *Am J Otolaryngol* 1992; 13: 363–5.

Salasche SJ, Bernstein G, Senkarik M. *Surgical Anatomy of the Skin*. Norwalk, Connecticut: Appleton & Lange, 1988.

4 Preoperative assessment of the patient

Although most of the procedures carried out by dermatological surgeons are of a superficial nature, it is best to take the approach that there is never really a truly minor operation. Life-threatening complications, such as anaphylaxis or severe allergic reaction, malignant hypertension, cardiac arrhythmia, bleeding problems or bacterial endocarditis rarely occur, and the likelihood of this happening can be greatly reduced by careful preoperative assessment of the patient, and by ensuring that proper precautions are taken. It is also worth considering, before commencing surgery, whether or not you will be available for the immediate postoperative period, to deal with any problems that may arise. If not, alternative arrangements should be made, to ensure that the patient can contact a doctor who understands the principles of the procedure that has been performed. It is far better to be able to reassure a patient with a minor concern, or to manage a postoperative complication early, than to allow matters to progress unresolved.

4.1 History

General health

Routine preoperative assessment of all candidates for surgery should include enquiry about the patient's general health, current medication, allergies to drugs and history of a bleeding tendency or problems associated with wound healing. On reviewing the cardiovascular system, it is important to ask specifically about hypertension, angina, arrhythmia or previous myocardial infarction. With regard to the respiratory system, a history of bronchial asthma, emphysema or chronic cough may indicate decreased respiratory function, which may cause a problem in patients who have to lie supine for long periods. A history of hepatitis or cirrhosis may indicate inability to cope with some drugs, particularly local anaesthetics, if used in large amounts. Enquiry about bleeding following laceration, dental treatment or other minor surgical procedures may bring to light thrombocytopenia or coagulation factor deficiencies. Serious haematological diatheses such as haemophilia are likely to be elicited from the history, but mild conditions such as von Willebrand's disease may not be recognised, and may present during skin surgery as failure of clotting.

Drug history

Patients should be asked what drugs they are taking; those on beta-blockers, monoamine oxidase inhibitors or tricyclic anti-depressants may be intolerant of vasoconstrictors used in conjunction with local anaesthetics. It is also important to ask specifically about drugs that may not be regarded as medication, such as cold remedies or preparations for headaches, which nevertheless contain aspirin. Since aspirin can affect the function of platelets during their lifetime, it is best to ask the patient to refrain from all aspirin-containing compounds for at least 1 week prior to surgery. Other non-steroidal anti-inflammatory drugs (e.g. indomethacin) appear to have less effect than aspirin on haemostasis. Anti-coagulant therapy can cause significant bleeding during extensive skin surgery; where possible, the anti-coagulant may need to be discontinued 2 days prior to surgery and for 24 h thereafter. If anti-coagulant therapy cannot be stopped, it is reasonable to postpone surgery until the prothrombin time does not exceed twice the control value. It is advisable to carry out the platelet count in patients on cytotoxic agents.

Drug allergy

Specific enquiry should be made as to allergy to systemic antibiotics, particularly penicillin, and to local anaesthetic agents. Patients should also be asked routinely about allergy to topical anaesthetics, antibacterial preparations containing iodine, topical antibiotics and surgical tape before they are applied to the skin.

The paediatric patient

It is essential that children are seen with their parents when surgery is being planned. It is often useful to provide parents with handwritten information regarding the nature of their children's surgery, as anxious parents may not retain much of what is said.

When performing surgery on a child every effort must be made to allay apprehension, fear and pain and to encourage the child's co-operation. It is essential to be truthful and, in some cases, it is useful to show the child the instruments that will be used and to demonstrate their use on a puppet or doll. Parents should always be offered the opportunity of staying with their children during surgery; a calm and positive parent can have a profoundly soothing effect during a surgical procedure. Older children may be relaxed by their favourite story book or song.

Risk of infection

Clearly, it is important to ask specifically about the presence of valvular or other structural heart disease, synthetic heart valves and/or a pacemaker. The prophylactic regimes for patients with these have been discussed in Chapter 2, Section 2.6. It may be prudent to commence a relevant topical antibiotic for infected lesions up to 1 week before surgery.

Of increasing importance to the dermatological surgeon is the possibility of contracting hepatitis B or HIV infection from patients. It is advisable for all those carrying out regular dermatological surgery to be immunised against hepatitis B. Regrettably, no such immunisation is currently available as a protection against HIV. It may, however, be possible to identify patients at an increased risk of carrying HIV, by asking about lifestyle, sexual habits or a history of multiple blood transfusion or intravenous drug abuse.

History of wound healing

It is wise before contemplating any dermatological surgery to assess the possibility of poor wound healing as evidenced by excessive scar formation following previous operations. The outcome of surgical scars is highly unpredictable, but are usually fine on the face and may become wide on the back or hypertrophic on the sternum and deltoid areas, or in those of dark skin. Keloid scarring most commonly occurs in patients aged 10–30 years, in black and Hispanic people, and may run in families. Some scars in children that become hypertrophic may eventually flatten, soften and fade with time. On the back, excision of lesions followed by allowing the wound to heal by secondary intention can sometimes lead to a better cosmetic scar, with less spreading of the scar than occurs when a wound has been sutured.

Wound healing has been shown to be much slower in people who smoke, and scars tend to be wider in smokers than non-smokers. Patients should be instructed to stop smoking particularly before graft and flap surgery where blood supply to the area may be reduced by smoking.

Wound healing in general may be adversely affected by drugs such as corticosteroids, anti-metabolites, immunosuppressive agents, penicillamine and colchicine, although this is not likely to pose a great problem in skin surgery.

4.2 Examination of the patient

All patients undergoing more advanced skin surgery should routinely have their blood pressure, heart rate and cardiovascular system checked. A rapid appraisal of the overall cardiovascular and respiratory system function is prudent, to determine a patient's tolerance to lying flat during the surgical procedure. The lesion for which surgery is going to be undertaken must be assessed; it should be measured and any ulceration recorded.

4.3 Laboratory evaluation

Ulcerated or infected lesions should be swabbed for microbiology, and an appropriate systemic or topical antibiotic may be indicated. It is not usually necessary to carry out other laboratory investigations before dermatological surgery. Patients with a history of bleeding problems or those who appear anaemic should have a complete full blood count including measurement of platelet count, a prothrombin time and partial thromboplastin time. It may be prudent to arrange for a preoperative electrocardiogram (ECG) in a patient with recent cardiac-type pain, to rule out the possibility of a recent myocardial infarction. Exceptionally, it may be necessary to carry out cryoglobulin and cold agglutinin tests, if these are felt to be clinically indicated, in patients undergoing extensive cryosurgery.

4.4 Preoperative photography

Photography is a very important adjunct to the preoperative assessment of the patient and should be carried out wherever possible. It enables complete documentation of the nature and site of the lesion, which may be helpful for medico-legal reasons, and is often useful later when the histol ogy proves to be more interesting than previously expected! In addition, preoperative photography allows more accurate assessment of the site of surgery at follow up.

For most purposes, a good quality 35 mm camera fitted with a zoom lens and an ordinary automatic flash is adequate. Some advocate use of a ring flash, which may be particularly useful for lesions in cavities such as the mouth. Film for slides is suitable for most purposes. Polaroid® systems have the advantage of enabling a photograph to be attached to the patient's records quickly, but are expensive. It is wise to take shots at several angles, and to bracket the focus and flash settings, to enable eventual selection of the best photograph.

4.5 Informed consent

The issue of informed consent is perhaps one of the most important aspects of dermatological surgery, especially in these more litigious times. Obtaining informed consent involves much more than the patient simply signing a form. Informed consent implies that the patient has been given sufficient information to enable an intelligent assessment of the potential benefits and disadvantages of the proposed therapy. The patient must be of sound mind and adult years; if the patient is legally a minor, then a parent or guardian must give written consent. In outlining the risks involved, it is important to give a full description in lay terms of the proposed procedure, and of any alternative approaches. It is essential that the surgeon be honest, and avoid giving any guarantees that cannot, at a later stage, be upheld. After discussion of the procedure, the patient should be asked if he or she has any questions regarding the information given, or if there are any aspects that have not been fully understood. At this stage, it is probably wise to obtain written consent from most patients. The consent form should be written using simple lay terms, and consent should be obtained personally by the surgeon.

It must be realised that the signing of a consent form by the patient is only an indication that the procedure has been discussed. Unfortunately, patients tend to remember the more favourable aspects of such discussions and tend to suppress the less favourable facts. It is therefore wise in certain circumstances to record in the notes exactly what information has been given to the patient, in case a legal action has to be defended at a later stage. There is no doubt that a fair number of malpractice claims have to be settled purely because of a lack of documentation in the notes as to what the patient was told.

4.6 Surgery during pregnancy

Skin surgery may be required during pregnancy, most often for changing naevi or pyogenic granulomas. Because of altered haemodynamic and anatomical factors, the pregnant patient is more susceptible to syncopal attacks. This tendency can be reduced by positioning the patient on her left side, thus reducing pressure from the uterus on pelvic muscles. In an acute hypotensive crisis, the supine Trendelenburg's position should be avoided, but venous return can be increased by elevating the legs.

When possible, surgery should be avoided during the first trimester and particularly during days 15 to 56 which is the period of organogenesis. Local anaesthetics are not regarded as teratogenic if used in nontoxic doses (Chapter 5). The concomitant use of adrenaline as a vasoconstrictor could theoretically cause uterine artery spasm, with resultant reduced placental perfusion, but this is unlikely to be significant for small surgical procedures.

Chlorhexidine is the antiseptic of choice, but both hexachlorophene and povidine iodine should be avoided. When postoperative analgesia is likely to be necessary, paracetamol should be suggested; in the unlikely event of an antiemetic being required, promethazine is a reasonable choice. Antibiotics that are safe during pregnancy include the penicillins, cephalosporins and erythromycin (but not its estolate salt). Amino-glycosides and tetracyclines should be avoided. Sun exposure to the scar should be avoided for 6 months after delivery and lactation, as this may accentuate the tendency for hyperpigmentation that occurs as a result of the hormonal influences of pregnancy.

4.7 Patients with unrealistic expectations

In the case of patients requesting surgery for benign lesions or cosmetic reasons, it is particularly important to obtain a good assessment of their psychological profile, which may take some time. Patients who are worried about very minimal skin lesions, who complain about previous medical care or who have an obsessive or perfectionist nature, are more likely to have unrealistic expectations, and to be dissatisfied with the final outcome of surgery. In such patients, it may not be wise to carry out the procedure. Sometimes, delaying the patient's decision to proceed with an operation until they have discussed it fully with their family may be helpful.

Bibliography

Gormley DE. Cutaneous surgery and the pregnant patient. *J Am Acad Dermatol* 1990; 23: 269–79.

Gross DA. On history-taking before surgery. *J Dermatol Surg Oncol* 1981; 7: 71–2.

Kraushar MF, Steinberg JA. Informed consent. Surrender or salvation? *Arch Ophthalmol* 1986; 104: 352–5.

Laurence C, Sakuntabhai A, Tiling-Grosse S. Effect of aspirin and nonsteroidal anti-inflammatory drug therapy on bleeding complications in dermatologic surgical patients. *J Am Acad Dermatol* 1994; 31: 988–92.

Leshin B, McCalmont TH. Preoperative evaluation of the surgical patient. *Dermatol Clin* 1990; 8: 787–94.

Leshin B, Whitaker DC, Swanson NA. An approach to patient assessment and preparation in cutaneous oncology. *J Am Acad Dermatol* 1988; 19: 1081–8.

Redden EM, Baker DC. Coping with the complexities of informed consent in dermatologic surgery. *J Dermatol Surg Oncol* 1984; 10: 111–15.

Sebben JE. Prophylactic antibiotics in cutaneous surgery. *J Dermatol Surg Oncol* 1985; 11: 901–6.

Wagner RF, Grande DJ, Feingold DS. Antibiotic prophylaxis against bacterial endo-carditis in patients undergoing dermatologic surgery. *Arch Dermatol* 1986; 122: 799–801.

Weimar VW, Ceilley RI, Goeken JA. Aggressive biologic behavior of basal and squamous cell cancers in patients with chronic lymphocytic leukemia or chronic lymphocytic lymphoma. *J Dermatol Surg Oncol* 1979; 5: 609–14.

5 Anaesthesia

The vast majority of cutaneous surgery is carried out under local anaesthesia; it is therefore essential for the skin surgeon to have a good knowledge of the available agents, as well as of their metabolism, physiology of action and potential side effects.

5.1 Mechanism of action of local anaesthetics

Local anaesthetics exert their effects through depression of excitation of nerve endings, or through inhibition of the conduction process in peripheral nerves. The influx of sodium ions into the axoplasm is essential for the initiation of an action potential, and subsequent propagation of an impulse signal along a nerve. Local anaesthetics reduce conduction in peripheral nerves by decreasing the permeability of ion channels to sodium ions, a form of inhibition termed non-depolarising nerve block.

5.2 Available agents

All local anaesthetics are amphipathic, in that they possess a lipophilic and a hydrophilic component at opposite ends of the molecule. The two ends of the molecule are joined by an intermediate hydrocarbon chain. This contains either an ester or amide linkage and allows classification into two groups (Table 5.1). The amid-linked group includes lignocaine, bupivacaine and prilocaine. The ester-linked group may be represented by procaine. The amide anaesthetics have a much lower incidence of toxic reactions compared to the esters, and are therefore the drugs of first choice for local anaesthesia. The amide local anaesthetics are primarily metabolised by microsomal enzymes in the liver, and therefore should be used with some caution in patients with severe liver disease or on beta-blocker therapy, which decreases blood flow to the liver. By contrast, the ester anaesthetics are hydrolysed in the plasma by the enzyme pseudo-cholinesterase. Patients with a rare genetic defect of this enzyme are unable to metabolise the ester-type local anaesthetics, and toxicity is therefore increased in such patients. It is worth having a range of anaesthetics from each group available, since if the usual amide anaesthetic agents cannot be used, then anaesthesia might be possible using an alternative ester type of drug. The properties of the local anaesthetic agents commonly used for anaesthesia are shown in Table 5.1.

Amide anaesthetics

The most commonly used local anaesthetics are of the amide type. The prototype drug is lignocaine, which has the advantage of a rapid onset of action; it has become the standard medium-duration anaesthetic agent.

Table 5.1 Currently available local anaesthetic agents.

Agent	Class	Concentrations available	Vasoconstrictor	Onset of action (min)	Duration of action		Upper safe dose		Comments and special precautions
					Without v/c* (min)	With v/c (min)	Without v/c	With v/c (mg)	
Lignocaine	Amide	0.5%, 1%, 2%	Adrenaline 1/50 000–1/200 000	Rapid (2–3)	30–120	60–400	(6.6 mg/kg) 200 mg	500	
Bupivacaine	Amide	0.25%, 0.5%, 0.75%	Adrenaline 1/200 000	Slow (6–8)	120–240	240–480	(1.3 mg/kg) 150 mg	150	For prolonged anaesthesia or for postoperative analgesia
Prilocaine	Amide	0.5%, 1%, 2%, 4% (3% with felypressin)	Felypressin 0.03 unit/ml or Adrenaline 1/200 000	Rapid (2–4)	30–120	60–400	(6 mg/kg) 400 mg	600	Contra-indications: idiopathic and congenital methaemoglobinaemia, anaemic states, cardiac or respiratory failure, patients on paracetamol
Mepivicaine	Amide	1%, 1.5%, 2%, 3%	Levonordefrin 1/200 000	Rapid (2)	30–120	60–400	(4.4 mg/kg) 350 mg	350	Slightly more rapid onset than lignocaine
Etidocaine	Amide	0.5%, 1%, 1.5%	Adrenaline 1/200 000	Rapid (2–3)	200	240–360	(8 mg/kg) 300 mg	400	Rapid onset, prolonged anaesthesia
Procaine	Ester	0.5%, 1%, 2%, 4%	Adrenaline 1/50 000–1/100 000	Slow (6–10)	15–30	30–90	(6 mg/kg) 500 mg	600	Potent vasodilator, drug of choice for reversal of accidental intra-arterial injection of vasoconstrictor. Relatively high incidence of allergy
Chloroprocaine	Ester	0.5%, 1%, 2%	Adrenaline 1/200 000	Slow (6–12)	30–45	45–60	(8.8 mg/kg) 800 mg	1000	Uncomfortable burning sensation on injection; short duration; extremely short plasma half-life

* v/c, vasoconstriction.

It is available in concentrations of 0.5%, 1% and 2%, either with or without added adrenaline as a vasoconstrictor. Anaesthesia is achieved within a few minutes of intradermal injection of lignocaine, although in the absence of adrenaline the maximum effect may not be achieved for up to 5 min. Lignocaine with adrenaline will provide local anaesthesia for between 60 and 120 min, which is usually long enough for most dermatological surgery. For surgery extending over longer periods, bupivacaine has the advantage of being a more potent local anaesthetic with a much longer duration of action of 4–8 h. The main disadvantage of this agent is its slow onset of action, with the maximum effect being delayed for up to 30 min. This disadvantage can be overcome by mixing bupivacaine with equal amounts of 2% lignocaine solution, in order to combine the rapid speed of onset of lignocaine anaesthesia with the extended duration of bupivacaine anaesthesia. The duration of anaesthesia can be extended further by addition of adrenaline as a vasoconstrictor. Bupivacaine is available in concentrations of 0.25%, 0.5% and 0.75%, with or without adrenaline.

Ester anaesthetics

Procaine is an anaesthetic agent of the ester type with a rapid onset of action but a short duration, and is available in concentrations of 0.5%, 1% and 2%, with or without adrenaline. It is hydrolysed in the body to para-amino benzoic acid (PABA), and should not be used in patients who are allergic to PABA. It can be used in patients where amide anaesthetic agents are contra-indicated.

5.3 Use of vasoconstrictors

Addition of a vasoconstrictor to a local anaesthetic solution results in decreased intra-operative bleeding, increases the duration of the anaesthetic and by retarding the absorption of the anaesthetic reduces the risk of systemic toxicity. Adrenaline is by far the most commonly used vasoconstrictor for local anaesthesia, and is supplied pre-mixed with local anaesthetic solutions in a range of concentrations from 1:50 000 to 1:500 000. We have found that adrenaline at 1:200 000 is effective for producing vasoconstriction and does not significantly increase the toxicity of local anaesthesia. As adrenaline is rapidly degraded by ultraviolet light, oxygen and alkaline pH, adrenaline-containing solutions are prepared at an acidic pH, with anti-oxidants to increase their shelf life. The acidic nature of the mixture is said to increase the stinging which accompanies injection of local anaesthetic. Since lignocaine is itself a vasodilator, the full vasoconstrictor effect of adrenaline, readily evident because of the blanching of the infiltrated skin, may take some 10–15 min to be achieved. A disadvantage of the use of adrenaline is that potential sources of postoperative bleeding and haematoma formation from cut blood vessels may not be visualised during the procedure, because of the intense vasoconstriction.

The use of adrenaline is contra-indicated in patients with phaeochromocytoma, hyperthyroidism, severe uncontrolled hypertension and cardiac disease. Other relative contra-indications include: known cardiac arrhythmia, pregnancy, or concomitant therapy with monoamine oxidase inhibitors, tricyclic anti-depressants or beta-blockers. For patients in this latter group, it may be possible to employ small amounts of local anaesthetic containing adrenaline, or to use more dilute concentrations of adrenaline, such as 1:300 000 or 1:400 000.

The adverse side effects of local anaesthesia attributable to vasoconstrictor agents include increased pain during administration, due to the acidic nature of the anaesthetic, and tissue necrosis. The use of adrenaline in areas supplied with end arteries such as the digits and penis, and during the construction of flaps, should be avoided because of the possibility of inducing tissue necrosis. This is particularly important in patients with known cardiovascular disease or other vasospastic conditions.

5.4 Toxicity of local anaesthetics

Local anaesthesia as practised during routine dermatological surgery is generally safe. However, toxicity may occur when high doses of anaesthetic are used, such as for extensive procedures, when planning of anaesthesia has been poor or when the patient is allergic to a local anaesthetic agent.

Allergy to local anaesthetics

True allergy to local anaesthetics, especially of the amide class, is rare, and accounts for less than 1% of all reactions encountered. Allergic reactions are usually of a type I immediate hypersensitivity nature, and may vary from mild urticaria to severe cardiorespiratory collapse. Patients who are allergic to the amide group of anaesthetics usually do not show cross-reactivity with the ester group of anaesthetics, unless they are allergic to one of the preservatives in the anaesthetic solution, such as parabens or sodium metabisulphite. It is difficult to distinguish by history alone true allergic reactions from the much more frequent psychogenic reactions. Testing for those who may be allergic to anaesthetic agents is best carried out by progressive challenge to the agents available, in an area fully prepared for resuscitation. Prick tests may first be carried out on the volar aspect of the forearm with the test solutions at a dilution of 1:10, accompanied by a positive (histamine) and negative (preservative-free saline) control. If no reaction is noted at 20 min, then intradermal injections of the agents may be carried out. Initially, 1 mm wheals of the agents, diluted 1:1000, are injected and if no reaction is observed in 15 min, the subcutaneous injections of 2 ml of the agents may be undertaken. If no reactions occur at any of these steps then it is reasonable to assume that the patient is not allergic to the agents tested.

In patients who are truly allergic to all types of local anaesthetic agent available, it is possible to use as an alternative the injectable preparation of an anti-histamine such as diphenhydramine, to which adrenaline 1:100 000 can be added as a vasoconstrictor; the disadvantage of this approach to local anaesthesia is that such agents produce pain on injection, have a short half-life and are sedative. Even intradermal injection of normal saline may produce sufficient temporary anaesthesia to enable rapid minor procedures such as shave biopsies to be carried out.

Toxic reactions to local anaesthetics

Toxic reactions to anaesthetics may occur when the recommended dosage is exceeded (Table 5.1), or as a result of relative overdosage in patients with impaired capacity to metabolise the anaesthetic agent, as with the amide anaesthetics in severe liver disease. The dose of anaesthetic agent administered can be calculated using the following formula: volume (ml) $\times$ % concentration $\times$ 10 = dose (mg). Early manifestations of central nervous system toxicity include circumoral numbness and tingling, lightheadedness, nausea and vomiting. These symptoms will occur at blood levels of 1–5 µg/ml of lignocaine. Nystagmus, slurred speech, hallucinations, muscle twitching and grand mal seizures may develop at higher blood levels of 5–8 µg/ml lignocaine. In the event of these symptoms, the patient should be placed in a supine position, and oxygen by mask and a slow intravenous (IV) injection of diazepam should be given.

The cardiovascular side effects of local anaesthesia are, of course, potentially even more serious, and may result from either the toxic side effects of the local anaesthetics themselves, or from the stimulatory effects of adrenaline. Local anaesthetics can induce vasodilatation and consequent hypotension, and may also depress myocardial contractility. With higher doses, atrial or ventricular block, or arrhythmias, may occur, leading to myocardial depression and cardiac arrest. Usually, the central nervous system side effects are obvious, and therefore the cardiovascular system effects can be avoided. However, anyone using local anaesthesia should be prepared to administer cardiopulmonary resuscitation if necessary.

Anaesthesia in childhood

General anaesthesia, even in a healthy child, carries a risk of mortality of 1 in 10 000 and this degree of anaesthesia is rarely required for dermatological procedures. Local anaesthetic agents have a narrow margin of safety in childhood and the dose should be accurately calculated on a milligram/kilogram body weight basis for each child. The maximum recommended dose of plain lignocaine is 3 mg/kg and thus for a 2% solution only 0.75 ml should be given to an infant weighing 5 kg.

5.5 Resuscitation measures

Adult emergencies in dermatological surgery

Treatment of anaphylaxis

In the case of an immediate anaphylactic reaction, administration of the causative agent should be stopped, if possible, and the patient made to lie flat. An intramuscular injection of 0.5–1.0 ml of 1:1000 solution of adrenaline should be given. The airway should be checked and oxygen given. Chlorpheniramine maleate, 10–20 mg, diluted in up to 5 ml water for injections, should be given slowly over 1 min IV. This may be followed by 4 mg orally every 6 h. Alternatively, 25–50 mg of hydroxyzine, or of diphenhydramine, may be given intramuscularly or orally every 6 h.

A combination of H_1 and H_2 histamine antagonists has been recommended as preferable in the prevention and treatment of anaphylaxis and anaphylactoid reactions, and cimetidine (300 mg IV 6-hourly) has been advocated in the treatment of anaphylaxis refractory to conventional therapy.

An IV infusion with 0.9% sodium chloride or 5% glucose should be set up. Blood pressure and pulse should be monitored. Hydrocortisone 250 mg IV should be injected immediately; the sodium phosphate form is preferable to the sodium succinate form for emergency use as it is already in solution form. This may be followed by 100 mg every 6 h IV, or oral prednisolone 40 mg daily for 3 days.

Where bronchospasm develops, aminophylline 250 mg IV over 5 min should be administered, followed by infusion of 250 mg in 500 ml 0.9% saline over 6 h. An alternative approach is to give nebulised terbutaline, salbutamol or metaproterenol (0.3 ml of a 5% solution of the latter in 2.5 ml of saline).

Endotracheal intubation may be necessary if laryngeal or glottic oedema with increasing stridor persists. In the case of hypotension, IV plasma or plasma expander should be given, with central venous pressure monitoring as necessary, since up to 25% plasma volume may leak into the extravascular compartment. Glucagon (1 mg in 1 L of aqueous dextrose solution at a rate of 5–15 ml/min) may be useful for refractory hypotension in patients taking beta-blockers. Myocardial depression with associated pulmonary oedema may develop as a rare complication of anaphylaxis; rapid colloid fluid replacement, cardiac inotropic drugs such as dobutamine (5–20 µg/kg per min), dopamine (2–20 µg/kg per min) or amrinone, with or without intra-aortic balloon pump therapy, in the intensive care unit are indicated.

Convulsions

In the case of convulsions, either from anaesthetic toxicity or epilepsy, the airway should be checked and oxygen given. Diazepam 10 mg can be given slowly by the IV route until the convulsions stop. The possibility of hypoglycaemia must also be considered, and if confirmed 50 ml of 50% glucose should be given by slow IV administration.

Cardiac arrest

The following measures should be instituted.
• Summon help.
• Place the patient on a firm surface.
• Try a blow to the praecordium.
• Clear the airway and apply artificial respiration (four quick breaths or Ambu-bag® with 100% oxygen).
• Apply external cardiac massage (15 chest compressions followed by two quick lung compressions).
• Establish an IV saline drip (give sodium bicarbonate 4.2% 150 ml stat and repeat after 10 min).
• If available, give an immediate direct current (DC) shock at 400 J.

- Connect electrocardiogram (ECG) monitor leads and determine ECG pattern.

  (a) Ventricular tachycardia: administer a 200–400 J shock and repeat if necessary. If there is no response, give lignocaine 100 mg IV and repeat the shock. If there is still no response, give adrenaline 1 ml of 1:1000 IV and calcium chloride 10 ml of a 10% solution IV. Then repeat DC shock after cardiac massage. If bradycardia is present, 5 mg of atropine, and 10% calcium chloride solution (3–4 ml IV) should be given.

  (b) Asystole: give a sharp blow on the chest. If there is no response, administer intracardiac adrenaline 1 ml of a 1:1000 solution and calcium chloride 10 ml of a 10% solution and continue cardiac massage and ventilation.

Once the patient is stable give lignocaine 100 mg IV over 2 min followed by a lignocaine infusion at 4 mg/min for 30 min, then at 2 mg/min.

- Continue oxygen 35% by mask; in the case of prolonged anoxia, inject dexamethasone 8 mg IV.

Hypotension

In the absence of hypovolaemia:
- give metaraminol 0.5–1 mg IV slowly IV over 2–3 min; *or*
- noradrenaline 1–2 mg in 500 mg 0.9% saline infused at rate to increase heart rate to 60 bpm.

  If hypovolaemic (e.g. excessive blood loss):
- establish infusion of 0.9% saline;
- take blood for group and cross-matching;
- establish infusion of colloid solution (e.g. Haemocel®).

Paediatric emergencies

Cardiac arrest

- Summon help.
- Clear airway.
- Maintain ventilation: mouth to mouth resuscitation.
- External cardiac massage (child on firm surface). Compress sternum with heel of hand 50–60 times per minute.
- Place drip and give sodium bicarbonate IV:

  (a) for infant 40 ml (20 mmol) sodium bicarbonate 4.2%;

  (b) for older children 60–80 ml (30–40 mmol) sodium bicarbonate 4.2%.
- Establish ECG oscilloscope.

  (a) If asystole give 2–3 ml of 1:10 000 adrenaline and 100–200 mg calcium chloride into heart BEFORE EXTERNAL SHOCK (see below).

  (b) If ventricular fibrillation: apply 50–70 J small infants; 100–250 J older children.

  (c) Resistant course fibrillation: lignocaine 10 mg or propranolol 1 mg IV before attempting DC shock with higher energy.

Status asthmaticus/anaphylaxis

- Give oxygen 35%.
- Aminophylline 4 mg/kg IV over 10 min

or adrenaline (1:1000 solution) intramuscularly or subcutaneously as follows:
    (a) 6–12 year old 0.5 ml;
    (b) 5 year old 0.4 ml;
    (c) 3–4 year old 0.3 ml;
    (d) 2 year old 0.2 ml;
    (e) 1 year old 0.1 ml;
    (f) under 1 year old 0.05 ml.
Repeat after 10 min if necessary.
    Also give the following.
- Hydrocortisone 100 mg IV stat.
- Chlorpheniramine 0.5 mg/kg stat IV.
- Followed with IV drip 5% dextrose at rate 70–120 ml/kg per day, with hydrocortisone 1.0 mg/kg per h and aminophylline 0.7 mg/kg per h.

Hypertensive crises

Diastolic blood pressure greater than 120 mmHg—diazoxide 5 mg/kg IV given and repeated according to response.

Convulsions

- Clear airway and administer oxygen (35%).
- Administer diazepam 0.25 mg/kg IV (below 1 year), 2.5 mg (1 year) to 5 mg (7 years).
- Consider hypoglycaemia, hypocalcaemia, hypomagnaesaemia. If prolonged anoxia give dexamethasone 4 mg IV followed by 4–8 mg intramuscularly daily for cerebral oedema.

Vomiting

Metoclopramide intramuscularly—1 mg (1 year), 5 mg (7 years).

5.6 Premedication

Some patients will be particularly anxious before surgery and may benefit from premedication, usually in the form of an oral benzodiazepine such as diazepam, taken at 2 h previously. Alternatively, where a patient is discovered to be very anxious immediately prior to surgery, rapid relaxation can be achieved by sublingual administration of diazepam; the patient being asked to suck 10 mg of the tablet placed under the tongue. This will usually relax the patient within 10–15 min. IV diazepam, which has the advantage of conferring amnesia for the procedure, is rarely required for dermatological surgery. Arrangements must be made in advance for a friend or relative to accompany patients given such premedication, to enable them to return home safely. Patients undergoing lengthy procedures may find music listened to by headphones particularly soothing and distracting.

Anxious children are probably best comforted by parents who, hopefully, will remain calm themselves. For infants and small children who require some form of preoperative sedation, chloral hydrate is one of the safest and widely used sedatives and can be administered in a dose of 75 mg/kg 30–60 min before the procedure, with a further 25–30 mg/kg being administered if the child is not showing signs of drowsiness 30 min after the first administration. Midazolam is a short-acting benzodiazepine which has the added advantage of inducing amnesia. It can be given in doses of 0.5–0.75 mg/kg usually orally and may be administered mixed with concentrated fruit juice for increased tolerance. For children over the age of 10 years, oral diazepam can be safely used.

5.7 Administration of local anaesthetic

It is recommended that gloves should be worn when inducing local anaesthesia. The anaesthetic may be given using a disposable syringe, and is best delivered using a 25-gauge needle which is available in 0.5 in or 1 in lengths. For anaesthesia prior to removal of small lesions, an insulin syringe incorporating an integral small bore needle is useful. An alternative system is to use a reusable dental syringe, into which can be loaded disposable cartridges containing local anaesthetic. The dental syringe needle screws onto the syringe barrel, and is therefore less likely to become detached, with resultant spraying of the patient and doctor; in addition, the bore of the needle is much narrower. Longer needles have the advantage that anaesthesia can be induced over a larger area with a smaller number of needle insertions. Should the size of the field to be anaesthetised necessitate withdrawal and reinsertion of the needle, it is preferable to reintroduce the needle through an area of skin that has already been anaesthetised. In the case of the palms or the soles, the needle may initially be inserted at the side of the foot underneath the palmar or plantar skin, and then moved progressively nearer the centre of the palm or sole through anaesthetised skin. Needles should be orientated with the bevel facing up to ensure that infiltration occurs at the level of the needle tip, and should be checked for patency before insertion into the skin. In order to make sure the needle has been placed extravascularly, aspiration should always precede injection, and the rate of injection during needle withdrawal should be slow.

Pain following intradermal injections of 1% lignocaine with adrenaline 1:100 000 may be significantly reduced by warming the solution to 37°C, with addition of sodium bicarbonate (50 mmol/l) sufficient to raise the pH to 7, the latter mixture remaining active for up to 1 week following its preparation.

In all cases, sufficient time should be allowed for anaesthesia to develop. Where adrenaline has been used it takes 5–8 min for full vasoconstriction and anaesthesia to develop. The surgeon should always confirm, using a sharp needle, that the relevant area of skin has been adequately anaesthetised before making an incision. Intradermal injection of local anaesthetic produces anaesthesia very quickly; injection into the subcutaneous fat results in delayed onset of anaesthesia but is less painful for the patient. Pain experienced by the patient can be lessened by injecting the local anaesthetic slowly, warming the anaesthetic to 37°C or by using the agent at weaker concentrations. In the case of small children, topical skin anaesthesia using an eutectic mixture of local anaesthetic (EMLA®) cream (see below) 2 h previously may decrease the pain of the injection. Alternatively, cooling of the skin with an ice pack, chilled soft drink or fluoroethyl spray may decrease the pain associated with the delivery of local anaesthetic.

A potential problem with infiltrative anaesthesia is the inevitable accompanying tissue distortion, which may render subsequent surgery more difficult. This problem can be lessened by injecting smaller amounts of anaesthetic, and by massaging the infiltrated area of skin before carrying out the surgery. It is appropriate to mark the planned incision lines in ink on the skin surface prior to infiltration of the anaesthetic.

A nitrous oxide–oxygen mixture for the relief of pain (as opposed to general anaesthesia) is a safe outpatient procedure. However, the oxygen concentration should never be allowed to fall below that found in air.

5.8 Field blocks

Field blocks are particularly useful when large areas of skin need to be anaesthetised, as on the scalp or ears, or in situations, such as the tip of the nose, where local infiltration may be painful, or where tissue distortion must be avoided (Fig. 5.1). The anaesthetic is injected around the base of the structure at the locations of the feeding nerves, thus avoiding multiple injections into the areas themselves.

5.9 Peripheral nerve blocks

Peripheral nerve blocks anaesthetise large areas of skin using small amounts of anaesthetic, avoid distortion of the surgical site and can often can be achieved with considerably less discomfort than that associated with infiltrative anaesthesia. A knowledge of the anatomy of the nerve is clearly essential. Temporary paralysis is not unusual when peripheral nerves are blocked with anaesthetic, and may last up to 1–2 h. Paraesthesiae may be induced if the nerve is punctured with the needle, and nerve damage may result if anaesthetic is injected with the needle in the nerve foramen. Other possible complications include intravascular injection with subsequent haematoma formation, and abscess formation around the nerve foramen, should the procedure not be carried out using a totally sterile technique. A brief description of the more commonly used nerve blocks follows.

Digital nerve block (ring block)

Each digit is innervated by pairs of dorsal and ventral nerves, as shown in Fig. 5.2. A digital block may be achieved with two injections of local anaesthetic at either side of the digit; it is commonly accepted that only anaesthetic without adrenaline should be used, but the risk of digital gangrene

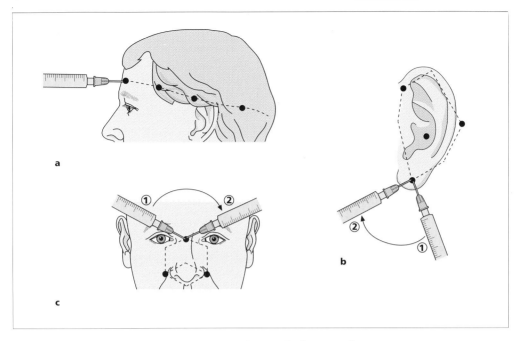

Fig. 5.1 Needle insertion points for field blocks for **a.** scalp; **b.** ear; and **c.** nose.

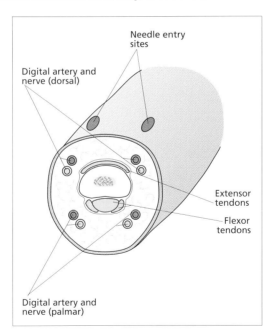

Fig. 5.2 Diagrammatic representation of digital nerves and needle entry sites for ring block of digit.

Needle entry sites

Digital artery and nerve (dorsal)

Extensor tendons

Flexor tendons

Digital artery and nerve (palmar)

has probably been exaggerated. The needle should be advanced towards the palmar digital surface, where approximately 0.5 ml of anaesthetic is deposited. It should then be partially withdrawn, and a further 0.5 ml of anaesthetic should be deposited at the dorsal nerve before removing the needle and repeating the injections on the other side of the digit. Failure to block the digital nerves is usually caused by placement of the anaesthetic too far away from the bone, alongside which the nerves lie. It is important to aspirate each time before injection, and not to inject more than 0.5 ml of anaesthetic. Larger volumes can cause obstruction of the end arteries as a result of vascular compression; this may be a particular risk when the digit is already oedematous, or in the presence of peripheral vascular disease.

A tourniquet will be required to control bleeding in the operative field during surgery, and should be placed following the digital nerve block. A rubber drain tube wrapped around the digit tightly enough to stop arterial blood flow, and secured using a pair of artery forceps, can safely be left in place for up to half an hour.

Infraorbital nerve block

Infraorbital nerve block provides anaesthesia to the lower eyelid, medial cheek, side of the nose and the upper lip. The infraorbital nerve emerges at the centre of the cheek from the intraorbital foramen, which is usually readily palpable about 1 cm below the infraorbital rim. The nerve block is probably best carried out through an intraoral approach (Fig. 5.3). With the middle finger of one hand over the infraorbital foramen, the thumb and index finger of the same hand are used to invert the upper lip. The needle is then inserted into the labial sulcus just behind the canine tooth, and advanced towards the pupil on the same side until it can be palpated just outside the foramen. Two to 3 ml of anaesthetic solution should then be deposited at this site; care should be taken not to enter the infraorbital foramen. Occasionally, a blood vessel in the area will be lacerated, giving rise to swelling and discoloration in the tissues around the orbit, which resolves in 2–10 days.

Mental nerve block

Mental nerve block is used to anaesthetise the lower lip and chin area. The mental foramen, from which the mental nerve emerges, can be palpated halfway between the upper and lower edges of the mandibular bone, below the second bicuspid tooth in the midpupillary line. The middle finger of

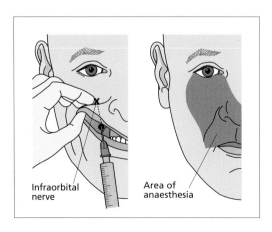

Infraorbital nerve

Area of anaesthesia

Fig. 5.3 Insertion of needle for infraorbital nerve block and area of anaesthesia.

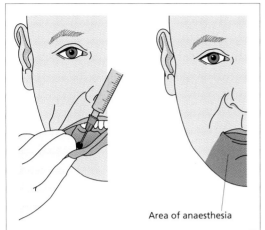

Fig. 5.4 Insertion of mental nerve block with area of anaesthesia.

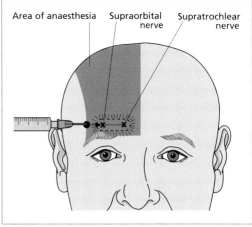

Fig. 5.5 Insertion of supraorbital and supratrochlear nerve blocks and area of anaesthesia.

one hand can be used to locate the foramen, with the thumb and forefinger everting the lip (Fig. 5.4). The nerve block can then be achieved by advancing the needle through the lower buccal sulcus below the second bicuspid, and injecting 1–2 ml of anaesthetic around the nerve.

Supraorbital and supratrochlear nerve blocks

These nerve blocks are useful for anaesthesia to the forehead and frontal scalp. The nerves emerge from the supraorbital and supratrochlear foramina, which can easily be palpated along the supraorbital margin in the mid-pupillary line and at the upper medial corner of the orbit, respectively. Regional anaesthesia may be induced by infiltrating local anaesthetic around the nerves at the level of the supraorbital notch, from the root of the nose medially to beyond the midpupillary line laterally (Fig. 5.5). Excessive quantities of anaesthetic solution may produce swelling of the upper eyelid, while haemorrhage may lead to peri-orbital swelling and bruising lasting up to 10 days.

Posterior tibial nerve block

The ankle block or posterior tibial nerve block is useful for surgery on the plantar surface of the foot, and is best performed with the patient prone. The posterior tibial nerve, which enters the foot at the ankle, innervates most of the plantar surface of the foot; only small portions of the medial and lateral foot surfaces are supplied by the saphenous and sural nerves, respectively. The posterior tibial nerve lies directly posterior to the posterior tibial artery and deep to the flexure retinaculum. The needle should be inserted at the level of the upper half of the medial malleolus, just posterior to the posterior tibial artery pulse and medial to the Achilles tendon (Fig. 5.6). It

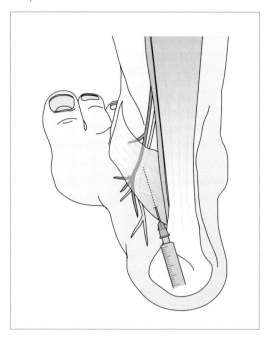

Fig. 5.6 Area of insertion of needle for posterior tibial nerve block.

should be advanced towards the posterior tibial surface until it touches bone; 3–4 ml of anaesthetic should then be injected following withdrawal of the needle by about 0.5 cm.

5.10 Tumescent anaesthesia

With the increasing use of liposuction in dermatological surgery came the necessity to anaesthetise larger areas of skin, especially at the level of the subcutaneous fat. It has been found that it is possible to use large volumes of very dilute local anaesthetics, injected into the subcutaneous fat, sufficient to give anaesthesia for liposuction, undermining and manipulation, although not for incisional surgery. Decreased toxicity, which has been noted as a feature of this technique, probably stems from a combination of factors including the relatively low vascularity of adipose tissue, lipophilic lignocaine being absorbed more into fat cells, and the lower concentration gradient between the solution and the bloodstream, thus reducing the rate of absorption.

Advantages of the tumescent technique include: (i) less bleeding in the subcutaneous tissue, perhaps as a result of the pressure of engorged fatty tissue with the large volumes of solution; (ii) long anaesthetic time (up to 16 h), reducing the need for postoperative analgesics; and (iii) the increased turgescence of the skin, allowing procedures such as dermabrasion to be carried out without the use of a cryogen.

Solution for tumescent anaesthesia

A typical solution for tumescent anaesthesia is as follows:
• 50 ml of 1% plain lignocaine;
• 1 ml of 1:1000 adrenaline;

- 12.5 ml of sodium bicarbonate (1 mmol/ml);
- 1 L of 0.9% sodium chloride in IV bag.

This will provide a solution of 0.05% lignocaine containing 1:1 000 000 adrenaline. If a solution of 0.1% lignocaine is required then a further 50 ml of 1% plain lignocaine can be added.

Delivery of tumescent anaesthesia

If excisional surgery is planned, then this should be undertaken using conventional local anaesthesia, using tumescent anaesthesia for the undermining and manipulation of large flaps. For relatively small areas, the use of a 3 in 25-gauge needle fitted to a 50 ml syringe may suffice. For larger areas, for example an abdomen for liposuction, then the 30 cm, 4 mm diameter Klein needle can be used, but some anaesthesia will usually be necessary for the needle entry point. For large volumes of injection, a refilling syringe fitted with a T-junction may be used, with one arm connected directly to the IV bag containing the anaesthetic solution.

It is important that the injection is undertaken slowly into the subcutaneous fat and that 20 min elapse before surgery commences. Typical solution volumes would be 150 ml for a cheek or chin, 750–2000 ml for a flank and 1000–2000 ml for lateral thighs or abdomen.

5.11 Topical anaesthesia

EMLA®

EMLA® is a topical anaesthetic cream produced by combining 2.5% lignocaine with 2.5% prilocaine. It should be applied to the relevant area under a plastic occlusive dressing for at least 2 h before the operative procedure. Used in this manner, EMLA® can provide effective anaesthesia for very minor skin surgery, such as removal of skin tags, curettage of molluscum contagiosum lesions, superficial cryotherapy and debridement of painful leg ulcers; EMLA® is also very helpful when used prior to venepuncture and infiltrative anaesthesia in children. It has been used to provide anaesthesia for patients undergoing superficial laser treatments, electrolysis and even split-skin grafting. However, it cannot provide anaesthesia below the level of the papillary dermis. It is suggested that EMLA® should not be used continuously on open wounds as it may impair defences against infection.

Mucosal anaesthetics

Topical anaesthetics available for mucosal surfaces such as the buccal and nasal mucosa include lignocaine, benzocaine and cocaine. Lignocaine at a concentration of between 2 and 5% is available in liquid, gel, ointment and spray form; anaesthesia can be achieved within about 15 min. Benzocaine is available in lozenge form. Cocaine, used in a 4% aqueous solution, has the unique property of being the only local anaesthetic that consistently produces vasoconstriction; its onset of action is usually within 1 min and its duration of action may be up to 2 h.

Ophthalmic anaesthetics

Amethocaine, used in concentrations of 0.5% or 1% for anaesthesia of the cornea and conjunctiva, has a short duration of action of 30–45 min. Anaesthesia of the eyelids can be achieved by first anaesthetising the surface conjunctiva; the rest of the eyelid may then be anaesthetised painlessly by introducing the needle through the anaesthetised area.

Adverse effects

Contact sensitisation is perhaps most common with the ester anaesthetic agent benzocaine, but can be a problem with lignocaine; it may also be caused by preservatives in the creams and topical solutions, such as parabens. Patch testing to the constituents of the topical anaesthetic preparation will be necessary to determine the causative agent.

Bibliography

Alonso PE, Rioja LF. Pain–temperature relation in the application of local anaesthetic. *Br J Plast Surg* 1993; 46: 76–8.

Barer MR, McAllen MK. Hypersensitivity to local anaesthetics: a direct challenge test with lignocaine for definite reaction. *Br Med J* 1982; 284: 1229–30.

Brueton MJ, Lortan JE, Morgan DJR, Sutters CA. Management of anaphylaxis. *Hosp Update* 1991; 17: 386–98.

Cohen SJ, Roenigk RK. Nerve blocks for cutaneous surgery on the foot. *J Dermatol Surg Oncol* 1991; 17: 527–34.

Committee on Drugs. Guidelines for monitoring and management of paediatric patients during and after sedation for diagnostic and therapeutic procedures. *Paediatrics* 1992; 89: 1010–15.

Curley RK, MacFarlane AW, King CM. Contact sensitivity to the amide anesthetics lidocaine, prilocaine and mepivacaine. *Arch Dermatol* 1986; 122: 924–6.

Dzubow LM. The interaction between propranolol and epinephrine as observed in patients undergoing Mohs surgery. *J Am Acad Dermatol* 1986; 15: 71–5.

European Resuscitation Council Basic Life Support Working Group. Guidelines for basic life support. *Br Med J* 1993; 306: 1587–9.

Fisher M McD, Graham R. Adverse responses to local anaesthetics. *Anaesth Intensive Care* 1984; 12: 325–7.

Foster CA, Aston SJ. Propranolol–epinephrine interaction: a potential disaster. *Plast Reconstr Surg* 1983; 72: 74–8.

Gilnert RJ, Zachary CB. Local anaesthetic allergy: its recognition and avoidance. *J Dermatol Surg Oncol* 1991; 17: 491–6.

Hanson GC. Resuscitation. In: Ogilvie C (ed.) *Birch's Emergencies in Medical Practice*, 11th edn. London: Churchill Livingstone, 1981: 309–17.

Juhlin L, Evers H. EMLA: a new topical anaesthetic. *Adv Dermatol* 1990; 5: 75–92.

Katz J. *Atlas of Regional Anesthesia*. Norwalk, Connecticut: Appleton-Century-Crofts, 1985.

Klein JA. Tumescent technique for local anaesthesia inproves safety in large-volume liposuction. *Plast Reconstr Surg* 1993; 92: 1085–98.

Long CC, Motley RJ, Holt J. Taking the 'sting' out of local anaesthetics. *Br J Dermatol* 1991; 125: 452–5.

Maloney JM. Nitrous oxide–oxygen analgesia in dermatologic surgery. *J Dermatol Surg Oncol* 1980; 6: 447–50.

Powell DM, Rodeheaver GT, Foresman PA. Damage to tissue defenses by EMLA® cream. *J Emerg Med* 1991; 9: 205–9.

Ruzicka T, Gerstmeier M, Przybilla B, Ring J. Allergies to local anaesthetics: comparison of patch test with prick test and intradermal test results. *J Am Acad Dermatol* 1987; 16: 1202–8.

Schatz M. Skin testing and incremental challenge in the evaluation of adverse reactions of local anaesthetics. *J Allergy Clin Immunol* 1984; 74: 606–16.

Sivers TD, Eyee JD, Foley ME *et al.* Midazolam for conscious sedation during paediatric oncology procedures: safety and recovery parameters. *Paediatrics* 1991; 88: 1172–9.

Smith NT, Miller RD, Corbascio AN (eds). *Drug Interaction in Anesthesia.* Philadelphia: Lea & Febiger, 1981.

Weber PJ, Weber M, Dzubow LM. Sedation for dermatologic surgery. *J Am Acad Dermatol* 1989; 20: 815–26.

Winton GB. Anesthesia for dermatologic surgery. *J Dermatol Surg Oncol* 1988; 14: 41–53.

Wood B. *A Paediatric Vade-Mecum.* London: Lloyd-Luke Ltd, 1977.

6 Sutures and suture techniques

6.1 Suture and closure materials

Suture materials may be arbitrarily designated as either absorbable or non-absorbable, with an absorbable suture being defined as one that has been absorbed within 60 days of implantation. Sutures can also be classified according to their physical characteristics as either single stranded (monofilament) or multifilamentous; the latter are usually braided. They can be further subdivided on the basis of being either synthetic (e.g. polypropylene, nylon and polydioxanone) or of natural origin (e.g. silk and catgut). All of these various properties have their advantages and disadvantages. For example, braided sutures are easy to tie, but the braiding increases their ability to harbour organisms, and also increases tissue reaction to the sutures. By contrast, the synthetic monofilament sutures generally have greater tensile strength and cause considerably less tissue reaction, but they are stiff and handle less well, are more difficult to tie and have a greater tendency to cut through tissue.

Suture memory, elasticity and plasticity

Suture memory refers to the tendency for a suture material to return to its original physical configuration during suturing. Thus, sutures with high memory are more difficult to tie and the knot is less secure, as the suture tends to untie to regain its former shape. Nylon sutures have a high memory, whereas silk is a suture material with low memory.

A suture's inherent tendency to regain its original form and length after stretching is referred to as elasticity, while plasticity refers to a suture material which on stretching retains its new length. Elasticity and plasticity become important where there is swelling of a wound. A suture with a high degree of plasticity will stretch and will tend not to cut through the swollen tissue. However, it will retain its stretched size after the wound swelling subsides, leading to a loose suture.

Absorbable sutures (Fig. 6.1)

Absorbable sutures are used for the closure of subcutaneous dead space and the approximation of wound edges, in order to minimise tissue distension during the wound healing process. Generally, they are placed in the dermis and are subsequently absorbed as part of the inflammatory response. Many synthetic absorbable sutures undergo degradation by hydrolysis which is much more predictable and consistent than the enzymatic digestion which occurred for catgut.

If absorbable sutures are placed too superficially they may not be absorbed as effectively, moreover, they have an increased tendency to be

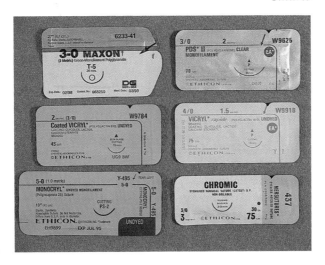

Fig. 6.1 Commonly used absorbable sutures.

eliminated from the wound, giving rise to a 'suture spit'. The majority of absorbable sutures are of the braided type.

Braided absorbable sutures

Polyglactin 190. Polyglactin 190 (Vicryl®) is a braided synthetic suture of high tensile strength, this being twice that of catgut. It is coated to facilitate tying, and can be purchased as either clear or blue-coloured thread. It is absorbed by hydrolysis, with 45% loss in strength in 14 days and 80% loss in 21 days. Although Vicryl® does provoke an inflammatory tissue response, this is less than with catgut or Dexon®. Vicryl® probably does not contribute much to wound strength after 40 days, and is completely hydrolysed at 60–90 days.

A new polyglactin 910 suture known as Vicryl *rapide*® has recently been produced. This suture has a lower molecular weight than coated Vicryl®, and is more rapidly hydrolysed than the original product, with its tensile strength being 50% by 5 days. The use for Vicryl *rapide*® would be in wounds where only short-term support is required (e.g. on the face).

Polyglycolic acid. Dexon® is a synthetic braided absorbable suture made of polyglycolic acid; it is available with a lubricated coat (Dexon Plus®), enabling it to slip through tissue and tie easily. It is degraded by hydrolysis; a significant decrease in its breaking strength to about one-third occurs by 30 days, and absorption is complete within 90–120 days.

Monofilament absorbable sutures

Polydioxanone. Polydioxanone is a synthetic monofilament absorbable suture, marketed as either PDS® or Maxon®. Because of its monofilament nature it has less tendency to harbour infection, although it is stiffer and more difficult to tie. The main advantage of polydioxanone as a suture material is that sutures retain significant breaking strength (60% tensile strength) at 4 weeks, and the time to complete hydrolysis and absorption is around 180 days. The high tensile strength and delayed absorption of this suture material enable the surgeon to minimise the likelihood of wound dehiscence in areas of tension and where there are large underlying muscles, such as on the upper chest and back.

Poliglecaprone 25. This is a new monofilament synthetic absorbable suture material produced as a copolymer of glycolide and caprolactone. It is marketed under the name Monocryl® and has a high initial tensile strength, being about double that of chromic catgut. It loses its tensile strength much more rapidly than PDS®, having lost some 50% of its strength by hydrolysis in 7 days. It is noticeably softer, more pliable and has greater tissue glide than braided sutures such as Vicryl® but, as with any monofilament suture, knots must be tied securely. It is presently supplied in an undyed form.

Catgut

Catgut is derived from the submucosa of the small intestine of sheep, or the serosal layer of the small intestine of cattle. Since catgut is a natural product, there is no uniformity of strength along the length of the suture, which may lead to development of weak spots. Treatment of catgut with chromium salts produces a tougher suture material known as chromic catgut which resists absorption to a greater degree than plain catgut, but absorption can be variable.

Catgut has been almost entirely superseded as a material for subcutaneous suturing by the newer materials discussed above, because of the degree of tissue reaction evoked, interbatch variation and the rapid decline in its tensile strength with time.

Non-absorbable sutures (Fig. 6.2)

Synthetic monofilament sutures

Nylon (Monofilament polyamide 6 and 66). Nylon, first introduced in the 1940s, is still widely used under the trade name of Ethilon®. Nylon sutures are stiff with a high memory and are therefore difficult to tie, but possess great tensile strength and evoke minimal tissue reaction, enabling them to remain in place for long periods. They have a smooth surface, which

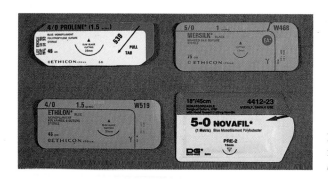

Fig. 6.2 Commonly used non-absorbable sutures

decreases bacterial colonisation. Monofilament nylon sutures are available as black, green or clear threads; green threads have the advantage of being easily distinguishable from hair in hair-bearing areas.

Polypropylene. Polypropylene (Prolene®) is a flexible monofilament suture with a tensile strength only slightly less than that of nylon. It has an extremely smooth surface, which results in very little drag during suture placement, and which enables the suture to be removed easily even several weeks after placement, as in the case of an intradermal running stitch. However, the extreme smoothness of polypropylene leads to lower knot security; should the wound swell after suture placement, the suture will be deformed and become loose when the wound swelling subsides.

Polybutesta. Polybutesta (Novafil®) is a recently introduced synthetic monofilament suture with a high tensile strength similar to that of nylon. However, it passes easily through tissue and has relatively little memory, making suture tying easy and knot security good. In addition, its elasticity ensures that sutures return to their original length following resolution of tissue oedema, resulting in continued apposition of wound margins.

Non-synthetic non-absorbable sutures

Silk. Silk is a natural fibre extruded from the silkworm. Braided silk (Mersilk®) is a suture that handles and ties well; its softness makes it very useful on mucous membranes such as the mouth and lips, where it is preferable to avoid bristly synthetic monofilament sutures. However, because of its braids, silk encourages infection, and provokes a marked inflammatory response, which may compromise the cosmetic result of surgery. In addition, removal from the skin can be painful, especially if sutures are left in longer than 4–5 days. For these reasons, silk is not often used for skin closure.

Range of suture diameter

Sutures are classified according to United States Pharmacopeia (USP) criteria, which specify the diameter of a given suture material necessary to produce a certain tensile strength. The smaller the cross-sectional diameter of the suture, the higher '0' number it is rated; for example, a 6/0 nylon suture is thinner than a 4/0 nylon suture. Because the USP size is not related to diameter but to suture strength, a 4/0 polypropylene suture will have a different cross-sectional diameter than a 4/0 catgut suture. In general, 5/0 or 6/0 sutures are used for skin closure on the face, while stronger 3/0 or 4/0 sutures may be required for skin closure on the trunk.

Surgical needles

Surgical needles are designed to lead suture material through tissue with minimal injury, and are made from high-quality stainless steel. They may be either straight or curved. Curved needles are either half of a circle, three-eighths of a circle or five-eighths of a circle in curvature (Fig. 6.3). The

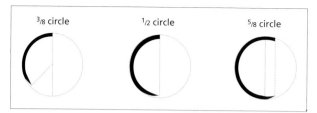

Fig. 6.3
Commonly used surgical needle shapes: three-eighths circle, half circle and five-eighths circle.

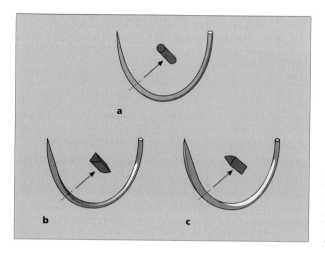

Fig. 6.4 Profile of surgical needles.
a. Round bodied;
b. cutting; and
c. reverse cutting.

three-eighths circle needle is the most commonly used; the half circle or five-eighths of a circle needle is sometimes useful in small cavities where the manoeuvrability of the needle is at a premium. Sutures with straight needles are useful for the placement of subcuticular stitches. The body of a needle may be either round or triangular in cross-section (Fig. 6.4); in the case of round needles, the body usually tapers gradually towards the point. In general, round-bodied needles tend to be used little in cutaneous surgery, but have the advantage of leaving a small hole that will not tear. The types of triangular needle most commonly used in cutaneous surgery are the reverse cutting and the conventional cutting needle (Fig. 6.4). The reverse cutting needle has its sharp cutting surface on the outside of its curvature, pointing away from the wound edge, and its flatter inner surface lying parallel to the wound margin. This results in considerably less tendency for tied sutures to tear through the tissue. By contrast, the conventional cutting needle has its cutting surface at the inner aspect of its curvature, facing the wound edge, which results in a greater tendency for tied sutures to cut through the tissue. The P needle (Ethicon®) has the same profile as cutting and reverse cutting needles, but the needle body is squarer in cross-section, which improves its resistance to bending when penetrating tough skin, and has sharp cutting edges. The slim blade needle (Ethicon®) is a delicate needle designed to provide a clean, smooth penetration desired for use on delicate tissues. It also has 'forceps flats' incorporated to ensure maximum stability in the suture holder. Ethicon® supplies most of its sutures in a one-step dispensing tray known as the Relay® system, which offers ease in needle attachment and suture delivery in an almost straight memory free way.

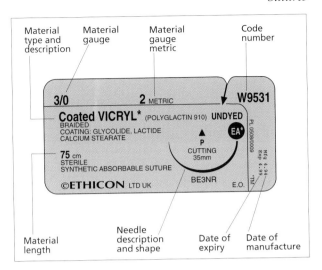

Material type and description — Material gauge — Material gauge metric — Code number

3/0 2 METRIC W9531

Coated VICRYL* (POLYGLACTIN 910) UNDYED
BRAIDED
COATING: GLYCOLIDE, LACTIDE
CALCIUM STEARATE
EA*
P
CUTTING
35mm
75 cm
STERILE
SYNTHETIC ABSORBABLE SUTURE
BE3NR
©ETHICON LTD UK E.O.

Material length — Needle description and shape — Date of expiry — Date of manufacture

Fig. 6.5 Features of needle and suture as described on package label.

The suture label

A typical suture package is shown in Fig. 6.5, together with an explanation of the main features of the suture contained within.

Choice of suture material

For the best cosmetic results, one should choose a non-reactive suture material, and a suture of the smallest diameter which will hold the wound together satisfactorily without tearing, such as a 5/0 or 6/0 monofilament material attached to a reverse cutting needle. Braided sutures should not be used in sites where increased infection is likely to occur, and subcutaneous sutures should be avoided altogether if a wound is deemed to be infected. Silk sutures should be used on the oral mucosa or genitalia, because they are less bristly and are therefore better tolerated by the patient.

Tissue reaction to sutures

Reactions to sutures occur partly as a result of tissue damage caused by passage of the needle and suture through the skin, and partly in response to the suture material itself. In the first few days after suture placement, there is usually a cellular infiltrate of polymorphs and lymphocytes around the suture; between the fourth and seventh days fibroblasts appear, and fibrous tissue deposition and chronic inflammation are evident around day seven. The reaction to sutures depends not only on the suture type, with braided sutures giving rise to more of an inflammatory response, but also on the amount of suture material placed in the wound. Subcutaneous knots may offer a haven for bacteria, and therefore the number of throws on a knot should be minimised in buried sutures. Re-epithelialisation may extend along the suture path, particularly with silk sutures, adding to the difficulty in their removal after periods of longer than 7 days. Allergy to suture material is rare but does occur with catgut; chromate-sensitive individuals may develop an allergic reaction to chromic catgut sutures.

Surgical staples

Surgical staples for wound closure can be placed faster than conventional sutures using a staple gun (Fig. 6.6), facilitate wound healing by everting wound edges and reduce the risk of infection since there is no suture track through the skin. Staples are particularly useful on hair-bearing areas such as the scalp, but on cosmetically important areas, such as the face, a better cosmetic result may be obtained using sutures. Staples are uncomfortable for most patients in intertriginous areas or on the back.

Tape closures

There are a variety of skin closure tapes (Steri-Strip®, Cover-Strip II®, Proxi-Strip®) available, which have excellent adhesive characteristics and are relatively non-occlusive (Fig. 6.7). A variation to the single tape closure is that of the Vari-Strip®, which comes as two separate components (Fig.

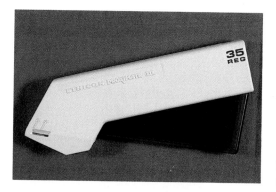

Fig. 6.6 Proximate® staple gun.

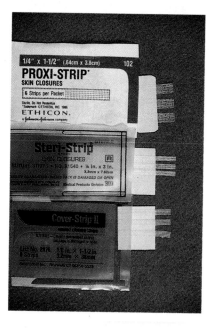

Fig. 6.7 Range of skin closure tapes.

6.8a,b). The two components of the strip are applied to either side of the wound and then the 'male' strip is fed through the 'female' component and the remaining adhesive liners are removed. The two strips are then pulled in opposite directions, until sufficient tension has been achieved to result in desired wound apposition. Suture tapes provide wound support for between 3 and 7 days. Their use avoids suture marks and can lessen the incidence of wound infection because skin puncture is unnecessary. Furthermore, skin tapes can be applied and reapplied to wounds for long periods after sutures have been removed, to provide continuing support to the wound edges and to minimise scar spreading. The skin surrounding the wound should be prepared by degreasing with alcohol and, after drying the skin, application of compound tincture of benzoin will help to secure the tape to the skin. Clearly, wounds that are under tension, or those that tend to invert, cannot be closed with skin tapes.

Tissue glues

Tissue glue is a relatively new wound closure material, available packaged in sealed ampoules (Histoacryl Blue®), and consisting of a preparation of monomeric *n*-butyl-2-cyanoacrylate, which polymerises quickly when in contact with tissue fluid (Fig. 6.9). The glue is coloured blue, so that the surgeon can readily see the sites of application. Instruments, clothes, swabs,

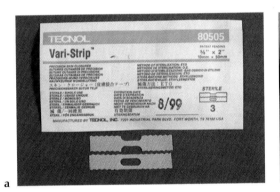
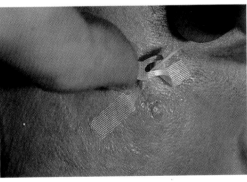

a   b

Fig. 6.8 a. Vari-strip® and **b**. application of Vari-strip® to wound.

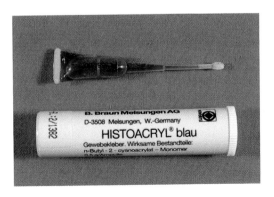

Fig. 6.9 Histoacryl Blue® tissue glue.

etc., coming in contact with the glue will adhere to it; instruments may be cleaned if necessary with dimethylformaldehyde or acetone.

The adhesive must be applied directly to the tissue edges, avoiding the depths of the wound to prevent delay in healing; the edges should be held apposed for about 1 min. Tissue glue is particularly useful in the closure of existing wounds in children since: (i) no local anaesthesia is necessary; (ii) a protective film across the wound decreases the risk of bacterial infection; and (iii) subsequent suture removal is avoided. Only wounds that are not under tension can be closed in this way; for wounds longer than 3 cm, it is recommended that the wound should also be secured by sutures.

6.2 Suturing techniques

Suture needles should be grasped by the needle holders in their middle third, to avoid bending the needle. The needle should enter the skin at an angle of 90°, pass through the dermis and subcutaneous tissue, and exit the wound again at 90° to the skin surface (Fig. 6.10). This will ensure eversion of the wound edges, which is usually considered to be advantageous, since with scar retraction depression of this area will occur. Handling of the wound margins should be done as atraumatically as possible, preferably by using skin hooks or toothed Adson's forceps. The size of the suture loop should be the smallest bite that opposes the wound edges; this usually means placing the suture within 1–3 mm of the wound edges. A wider bite may be required if the skin is under tension; if the tissue is thin, the needle may need to be inserted closer to the wound edges.

Tying the square knot

Fundamental to all suturing techniques is the ability to tie a square knot, which holds even with the newer monofilament sutures. The process of tying a square knot is shown diagrammatically in Fig. 6.11. The needle is first inserted and then pulled through the wound with the majority of the suture length following it. The long end of the suture is looped twice clockwise around a needle holder held in the closed position, which is then slightly opened and used to grasp the short end of the suture. Some surgeons would use only a single loop at this stage, for example during closure of thin skin as on the face or genitalia. The short end of the suture is now pulled through the loops of the long end of the suture, the surgeon crosses his or her hands over the wound, and next pulls the double loops

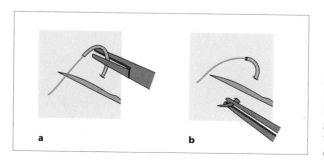

Fig. 6.10 a. Insertion of needle into skin and **b.** grasping of needle tip on opposite side of wound.

a   b

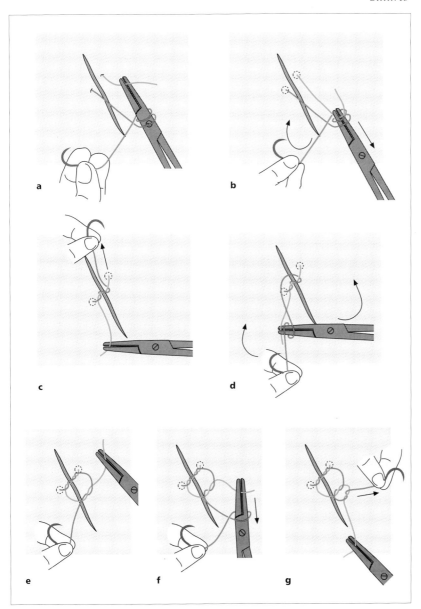

Fig. 6.11 a. Looping of suture over needle holder. **b.** Pulling of free end of suture through loop created in step **a** and towards surgeon. **c.** Suture is pulled taut across the line of the wound. **d.** Suture end attached to needle and far side of wound is looped over needle holder and free end is grasped. **e.** Free end of suture is pulled through the loop and away from the surgeon. **f.** Knot is completed by pulling free end of suture towards surgeon through final loop of needle end of suture and **g.** the square knot is tightened on to the skin surface.

onto the skin surface. It is important to realise that the knot should be secure but not tight at this stage, as a tight knot strangulates the blood supply to the wound edges. The short end of the suture is then released, and the long end of the suture is again looped around the needle holder, this time in an anti-clockwise direction. The needle holder is brought across the wound towards the short end of the suture, which is grasped and pulled through the loop, leaving the long end of the suture at the opposite side of the wound. As the final stage in the construction of the knot, the long end of the suture is looped once clockwise around the needle holder, which is then used to pull the short end of the suture through the loop. Occasionally, it may be necessary to place a further single or double loop to secure the square knot, if there is significant tension during wound closure.

Interrupted sutures

Once the needle exits the wound, the skin suture is completed using the square knot on the skin surface (Fig. 6.12). If necessary, while placing interrupted sutures the needle can be inserted through one edge of the wound, brought out of the centre of the wound and then reinserted to encompass the other side of the wound. It is important that the tract of the suture is symmetrical across the wound edges, as if it is asymmetrical it will result in overlapping skin edges.

The number of sutures will depend, to some degree, on skin tension and also on the number required to hold the wound edges in direct apposition. The knot should be placed to one side of the incision line after it is tied (Fig. 6.12) as this prevents the cut ends from getting caught in the wound, and it is also best to keep knots away from the wound as they tend to harbour infection. It is controversial as to whether one should start tying the knots in the centre rather than at either end of the wound. If there is a slight difference in the length of the wound margins, it is often best to start in the centre and decrease the difference in skin lengths by using the rule of halves (see Chapter 20). If there is tension in the wound closure, sutures can often approximate the edges best if started at the ends of the wound,

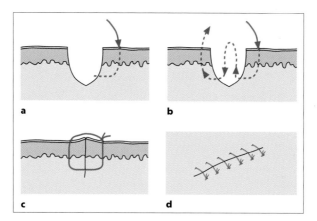

Fig. 6.12 Correct passage of needle through the skin. **a.** Entry perpendicular to the skin surface. **b.** Exit through base of wound and entry through base of wound at other side with needle exit perpendicular to the skin. **c.** Square knot tied on the surface. **d.** Knots on one side of wound.

with additional sutures in the centre of the wound being placed closer together.

The most frequently used suture is the interrupted simple skin suture. It has the advantages of simplicity coupled with the fact that if a haematoma or infection develops in the wound, it may be possible to deal with the complication by removing only one or two sutures, leaving the rest of the wound intact. It is, however, a relatively slow means of skin closure and for longer wounds a running cutaneous or subcutaneous suture may allow faster wound closure.

Buried interrupted sutures

Buried subcutaneous sutures are generally placed to collapse dead space, to approximate wound edges in order to eliminate tension and to provide continuing support to the wound when the superficial skin sutures have been removed. However, care should be exercised when trying to eliminate dead space, as too many sutures can lead to increased tissue necrosis and infection, and sutures placed in the fat layers usually lead to little if any tensile strength. It is best to place buried sutures so that much or most of the loop is in the dermis with some also in the subcutaneous fat (Fig. 6.13). It is important that the knot of a buried suture is at the bottom of the wound, so that it does not interfere with wound healing. The stitch is started deep in the wound, beneath the dermis, passing vertically upwards into the dermis and exiting through the dermis, across the wound and into the opposite dermis. After ensuring that both the leading and trailing suture ends protrude deep and to the same side of the wound, the suture is tightened and tied. It is usually best to tie the knot using the square knot, and if there is significant wound tension, it may be best to have an assistant hold the wound together, while tying down the first few subcutaneous sutures. The most common suture material used for this type of suture will be Vicryl®, or if stronger material is required, polydioxanone sulphate

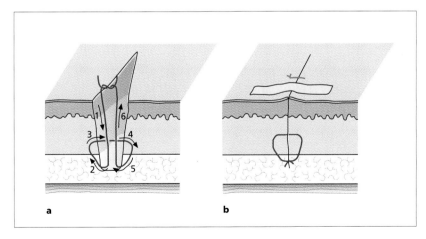

Fig. 6.13 a. Pathway of suture for a buried subcutaneous suture and **b.** with knot tied at the deep aspect of the wound.

(PDS®). The number of throws on the knot should be kept to a minimum and the suture cut 1 mm or less away from the knot to minimise the amount of foreign material placed in the wound.

When suturing wounds under some tension, it is often best to reduce tension by inserting buried interrupted sutures to the fascia where tissues are strongest and can best sustain tension.

Frequently, the placement of multiple buried subcutaneous sutures can be difficult during the closure of small surgical defects, because of the limited working space, which becomes progressively less with the tying of each buried suture. This problem may be overcome by delaying the tying of the subcutaneous sutures until all of the sutures have been placed, at which time the sutures may be pulled closed and tied with ease.

Dermal buried pulley suture

The dermal buried pulley suture has recently been described as a means of overcoming wounds with a moderate amount of tension. It consists of two continuous dermal sutures side by side. The first loop of this suture is placed as for the buried interrupted suture just described. Then, instead of just tying the knot, the procedure is repeated, the loop of the second adjacent dermal suture being placed approximately 2–3 mm from the first. After ensuring that both the leading and trailing suture ends protrude deep and to the same side of the pulley system, the suture is tightened by placing the first throw of the knot and lifting the suture ends and gently rocking them back and forth in a direction perpendicular to the wound, thus ensuring tightening of both loops of the buried dermal pulley system. The knot is then completed in the usual fashion.

Vertical mattress suture

The vertical mattress suture is specifically designed to cause eversion of the epidermal wound edges, collapse dead space and reduce tension (Fig. 6.14). It is the optimal suture for wound closure when eversion of the wound edges is required.

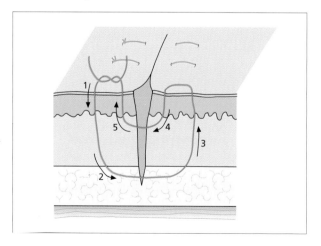

Fig. 6.14 Path of suture through the wound to create a vertical mattress suture.

To place a vertical mattress suture the first pass of the suture is identical to that of the simple interrupted suture except that the points of insertion and exit are some 5–10 mm away from the wound edge. After a simple interrupted suture has been inserted, the wound is re-entered on the same side as the previous exit site, close to the wound edge, exiting through the dermis, crossing the wound and exiting through the opposite wound edge, close to the wound, where the knot is tied. As a greater amount of the suture goes through to the dermal tissue, vertical mattress sutures give greater support to the wound than simple interrupted sutures. Because of this they also tend to restrict blood supply more than interrupted sutures, especially if tied under tension. If the suture is being used to relieve tension or to evert the wound it may be necessary to use only a few vertical mattress sutures in combination with simple interrupted sutures, which have generally been used to close the wound.

Half-buried mattress sutures

Half-buried mattress sutures are useful for closure of wounds where avoiding the compromise of vascular supply is important, such as in the closure of flaps, and also in reducing the effects of suture tracts (Fig. 6.15). The suture is placed by inserting and advancing the suture needle down to the level of the deep dermis or subcutaneous fat (unburied side), crossing the wound and entering the dermis or fat on the same level on the other side. The needle is then turned such that the suture tract becomes more superficial (but does not exit the dermis on the unburied side), before again crossing the wound, this time in the superficial dermis; the needle exits the epidermis before reaching the entry point, and the suture is then tied on the skin surface. Thus, on the buried side, a buried intradermal pass is made without the suture exiting the epidermis on that side.

Horizontal mattress sutures

The horizontal mattress suture is most useful for relieving wound tension, especially when this is great, and also acts to close dead space (Fig. 6.16). The suture begins at a distance away from the wound margin; the greater the amount of skin tension anticipated, the greater this distance should be.

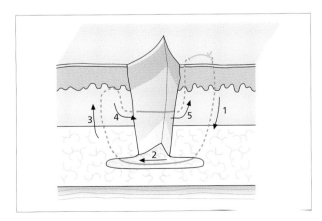

Fig. 6.15 Path of suture through the wound to create a half-buried mattress suture.

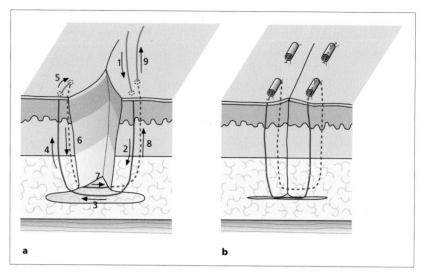

Fig. 6.16 Path of suture through the wound to create a horizontal mattress suture.

After passing through the skin, as in an interrupted simple suture, the suture course is parallel to the skin wound for 3–4 mm before re-entering the skin, passing through the dermis and the wound and exiting through the other side of the wound where it is tied. If there is a lot of tension this can lead to suture marks which to some extent can be reduced by the use of bolsters, made from dental rolls or flat buttons, which are used to distribute the tension on the skin. Problems with the horizontal mattress suture include strangulation of the tissue and crimping of the epidermis. It may be best to use simple continuous interrupted sutures to approximate the wound edges and rely on only relatively few horizontal mattress sutures to relieve skin tension.

Tip stitch and corner stitch

Tip stitches can be used to secure tips of tissue into corners without causing strangulation of the tissue (Fig. 6.17).

The suture is commenced by penetrating the skin 3–4 mm from the wound margin on the side away from the tip. When the needle exits the

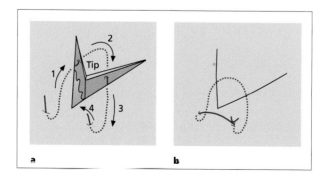

Fig. 6.17 a. Path of suture in tip stitch with **b.** square knot on skin surface.

dermis it is immediately passed horizontally through the wound, continuing through the same dermal plane of the triangular skin tip, then again crossing the wound and returning close to the site of entry on the other side of the wound, where it exits the skin and is tied. It is essential that the suture be placed at the same level in the dermis throughout its tract, travelling horizontally through the skin tip, and that when the suture is tied there is minimal tension on the tip, thus avoiding tip necrosis. When more than one tip exists this simple three-point suture is extended with the suture passing through the other tips of tissue to exit in a similar fashion as for the single-tip suture.

Continuous sutures

Continuous sutures for skin closure have the advantages of being fast to insert and of distributing tension equally along the course of the suture. They have, however, the disadvantages of not allowing fine adjustments at the end of suturing, and also of producing less exact approximation of the wound edges than with interrupted sutures. Furthermore, if sutures have to be removed because of infection or haematoma, the whole wound has to be opened, which is in contrast to the situation where interrupted sutures are present.

Running continuous sutures

For this suture, a simple interrupted suture is tied at one end of the wound, and the end with the needle attached is not cut. Sutures then continue looping continuously over and through the wound until the wound edge is closed and a square knot tied between the end of the suture and the last loop (Fig. 6.18). This suture allows quick skin closure, but is only recommended if the wound closure is not under significant tension.

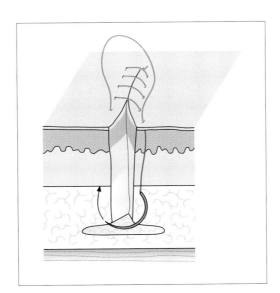

Fig. 6.18 Running cutaneous suture with square knot at beginning of suture.

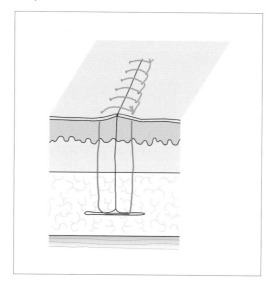

Fig. 6.19 The running locked (blanket) suture tied with a square knot at the beginning of the suture and a square knot on the last loop of the suture at its end.

Running locked suture

The running locked suture (blanket suture) is a variation of the simple running suture, the difference being that on each pass the suture is drawn through the previous loop and completed by tying it back on itself with a secure knot (Fig. 6.19). The running locked suture may be helpful where there is a lot of wound tension. It does have a tendency to leave ugly suture tracts and tends to reduce blood supply more than a simple continuous suture does, and should thus be used cautiously when blood supply is impaired.

Running horizontal suture

The running horizontal suture is a modification of the horizontal mattress suture previously described. After the suture is secured at one end, with a simple interrupted stitch, the leading end continues to make adjacent horizontal mattress passes without further ties until the distal end of the wound is reached (Fig. 6.20). It is important while making this stitch that each horizontal component be of the same length and distance from the wound margins as the others. It has the advantage of being a fast suture, which allows wounds of moderate tension to be closed with slight eversion of the skin edges.

Running subcuticular suture

The running subcuticular suture (Fig. 6.21) is an important suture as it leaves a highly cosmetic scar, free from the marks of suture punctures and suture tracts. In addition, this suture, when performed using monofilament sutures, can be left in place for weeks, adding support to the wound while minimising the possibility of suture tracts. The running subcuticular suture, however, cannot be used when there is much tension in the wound and is probably the most difficult of the continuous sutures to master. The suture

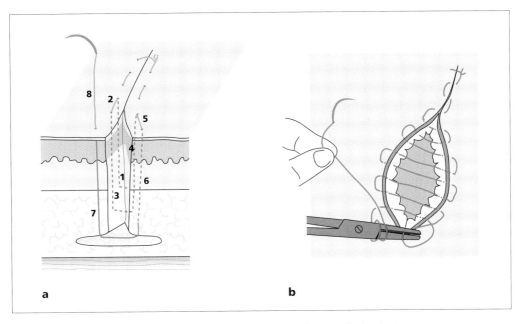

Fig. 6.20 a, b. Running horizontal suture tied with a square knot at the beginning, and a square knot on the last loop of the suture at its end.

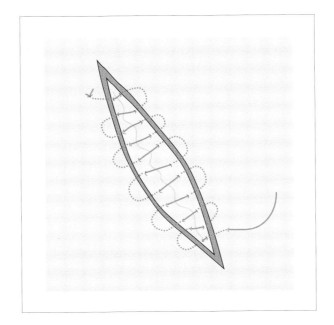

Fig. 6.21 The running subcuticular suture tied with a square knot at its beginning.

is started at one end by penetrating the skin, at which stage a knot can be inserted in the skin, or the free end can be held in place either by using skin tape or by a lead shot tied to the end.

The suture then begins at one end of the incision, with the needle entering through the apex of the wound. The needle is passed horizontally through the mid-dermis, grabbing a horizontal loop of one side of the wound and exiting into the wound, where a second pass is initiated at the same level in the dermis at the opposite side of the wound. The second pass does not start directly opposite the first, but instead is brought back about one-third of the distance from the first loop, grabbing a horizontal loop of similar length to the first. The wound is thus gradually closed with subsequent overlapping passes. When the other end is reached the wound is exited through the apex. It is then possible to tie off the other end of the stitch after the tension on the suture has been made to give the best closure without crimping. The entrance and exit points should be on the same side of the wound, the tension in the wound thus being along the straight line between these points.

The best suture material for this type of suture is polypropylene (Prolene®), as it has a low coefficient of friction and allows easy placement and removal of the suture, which can be left in place for 1–3 weeks, depending on the site.

6.3 The retraction suture

Good surgical technique requires adequate visualisation of the tissues being operated on, together with stabilisation of the surgical field. To some degree this may be achieved using the retraction suture, which is a simple untied stitch, which when held under tension by an assistant, can be used to pull skin out of the field of vision while creating a counterforce, and this has the effect of stabilising the surgical site.

For example, when removing a skin cyst, a suture may be placed in the skin ellipse created over the cyst and retraction achieved by pulling the suture tails, left long for this purpose. Tension may be directed to a different side or direction quickly by moving the direction of pull on the suture. Other uses include nail surgery for reflecting the proximal nail fold (Fig. 6.22), earlobe surgery or surgery in difficult anatomical sites, including the tongue, lip and eyelids. The retraction suture is probably best provided by a

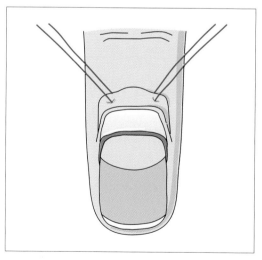

Fig. 6.22 Retraction sutures holding back proximal nail fold during nail surgery.

Table 6.1 Times for suture removal.

Area	Time to suture removal (days)
Eyelid	3–5
Face	4–7
Trunk	7–14
Extremities	7–14

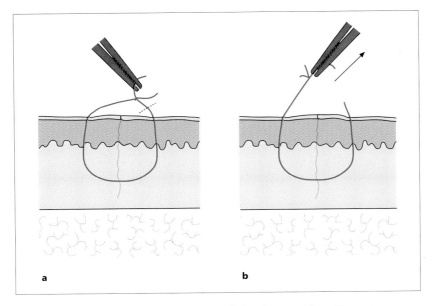

a   b

Fig. 6.23 Suture removal. **a**. Cutting suture below knot and **b**. pulling suture across the line of the wound.

3/0 or 4/0 non-absorbable suture, placed with a large skin bite, in order to cope with the tension which may be required.

6.4 Suture removal techniques

For removing sutures (Table 6.1), the wound should be thoroughly cleaned with an antiseptic. The suture can then be lifted slightly by holding one of the tails in a forceps, and using fine scissors, a No. 11 blade or suture cutting blade, the suture is cut beneath the knot. A hypodermic needle may be used to cut off fine sutures. After the suture is cut, it should be pulled across the wound, as pulling away from the wound may cause wound dehiscence (Fig. 6.23).

Bibliography

Ashall G. Atraumatic removal of microsutures. *Br J Plast Surg* 1991; 44: 238.
Bennett RG. Selection of wound closure materials. *J Am Acad Dermatol* 1988; 18: 619–37.

Campbell JP, Swanson NA. The use of staples in dermatologic surgery. *J Dermatol Surg Oncol* 1982; 8: 680–90.

Giandoni MB, Grabski WJ. Surgical pearl: the dermal buried pulley suture. *J Am Acad Dermatol* 1994; 30: 1012–13.

Lang PG. The partial closure. *J Dermatol Surg Oncol* 1985; 11: 966–9.

Ramsey ML, Marks VJ, Neltner SA. Surgical pearl: Delayed knot placement facilitates small wound closure. *J Am Acad Dermatol* 1996; 34: 137–8.

Salasche ST, Orengo I. Surgical pearl: the retraction suture. *J Am Acad Dermatol* 1994; 30: 118–20.

Snow SN, Dortzbach R, Moyer D. Managing common suturing problems. *J Dermatol Surg Oncol* 1991; 17: 502–8.

7 Electrosurgical devices and cautery

7.1 Principles of electrosurgery

Electrosurgery refers to the use of electrical currents in the controlled destruction of tissue. A widely used method of tissue destruction is that of cautery, which uses the heat generated from the conversion of a current passing through a metal tip to destroy tissue. Other electrosurgical units utilise high-frequency currents to destroy or cut tissue. In many instances they offer a simple yet cheap alternative to lasers, and may be used in different ways. In electrofulguration, a high-frequency, high-voltage, low-amperage current is delivered through the active electrode to the tip, which is not held in contact with the skin surface, but at a short distance above it. This results in an electrode–tissue air gap, with a spark resulting in superficial dehydration of the tissue. In electrodesiccation, a similar type of current is used, but in this case the active electrode tip is held in contact with the skin and the spark produced is finer than that in electrofulguration. Both electrofulguration and electrodesiccation are carried out by monoterminal electrosurgical units. For electrocoagulation, a bipolar low-voltage, high-amperage system is used, and tissue destruction is greater than with electrodesiccation because the current is greater. Furthermore, if the electrode tip is not in contact with the tissue, the current reaches the tissue by means of convection sparks and the coagulation is superficial, while if the electrode tip is in contact with the tissue, heat is produced and the tissues are deeply coagulated. Electrosection is another form of low-voltage, high-amperage, high-frequency electrosurgical current, which differs from electrocoagulation in being undamped and continuous. This allows the movement of an electrode through the tissue, vaporising cells as it passes but causing little tissue damage in the surrounding tissue. Thus, tissue may be cut while small vessels are coagulated, with minimal tissue damage in the wound or the tissue being removed.

During electrosurgery, there is a tendency for coagulated tissue to adhere to the tip, which makes the tissue sparking less effective. It is therefore helpful to clean the electrode frequently during surgery. The high-frequency electric current in the electrode tip is such that sterility is probably ensured. However, a sterile tip should be used for each patient, and tips should be either autoclaved or discarded following use on any particular patient.

Grounding

Grounding, when necessary, is performed using a dispersal plate, which allows the return of current to the electrosurgical device. When a high-frequency alternating current is applied, grounding is not required as electrical energy is alternately entering and leaving the patient. If the voltage is high and current low, then a grounding plate is similarly not required, for example when using a hyfrecator. In cutting modes, where high voltages and currents are used, a dispersal plate is required.

7.2 The hyfrecator

The hyfrecator is a high-frequency electrosurgical unit which produces a low-voltage spark resulting in the minimum formation of heat. It is frequently used in its monopolar form for electrodesiccation and electrofulguration, and for these purposes the patient does not need to have a ground plate attached. For electrodesiccation, the electrode tip is placed in contact with the tissue, while for electrofulguration the active electrode is held a few millimetres above the tissue and sparking occurs from the needle tip to the skin. High cure rates can be achieved for basal cell carcinomas with curettage and electrodesiccation. Other small lesions like warts can be treated by electrodesiccation, and telangiectasia by means of gentle electrodesiccation.

A wide range of tips is available for the hyfrecator including fine wire, ball and loop attachments. The most widely used electrode is the short-angled needle, which can be either non-sterile or individually wrapped in a sterile package. If the unipolar mode of the hyfrecator is being used in a sterile field, the handle of the hyfrecator can be kept sterile inside a sterile piece of tubing or sterile sleeve, or by using a sterile glove.

The hyfrecator also has a bipolar mode, which allows electrocoagulation of tissue through the use of bipolar forceps. This is suitable for the coagulation of small blood vessels during skin surgery. The hyfrecator has the disadvantage of not possessing an electrocutting mode.

7.3 Solid state and triode tube (electrosectioning units)

Solid-state electrosurgical units (e.g. Ellman®) have the advantage of not only producing electrodesiccation and electrocoagulation but also allowing electrosectioning of tissue. For electrodesiccation, electrocoagulation and electrosection a unipolar lead is used in conjunction with an active electrode, while the patient has a return plate (dispersion plate) attached to their skin. The 'cutting current' allows for microsmooth cutting of tissue with little heat formation, while also providing electrocoagulation. This ensures a relatively atraumatic technique, with little eschar production, thus reducing the fibrous scarring in wounds. A variety of electrodes are available, from straight wire electrodes for tissue cutting to loop type electrodes for paring or sculpturing tissue. Fine insulated electrode needles are available for the treatment of telangiectasia, and a hand piece allows the use of scalpel blades for electrosection, excisional surgery or for sculpturing tissue as in the treatment of rhinophyma. In addition, bipolar forceps are available for electrocoagulation of small-bore blood vessels.

Electrosurgery and pacemakers

High-frequency electrosurgical devices can interfere with certain types of pacemaker, and in particular cause inhibition of demand pacemakers. Fixed rate pacemakers, by contrast, are not interfered with by the electromagnetic radiation from this type of electrosurgical unit. If possible, electrosurgery using high-frequency surgical units should be avoided in patients with demand pacemakers, since electrocautery is a safe alternative. If high-frequency units are to be used in someone with a demand pacemaker, then the bursts should be kept short (less than 5 s) and the patient should be monitored by an electrocardiogram (ECG) oscilloscope during surgery.

Burns

If the dispersion plate electrode is not in sufficient contact with the patient's skin, then a high current can pass through a small area of skin resulting in a skin burn. In addition, electrosurgical units can cause the ignition of volatile agents such as ethyl chloride or alcoholic solutions of antiseptics, which should not be used in their vicinity.

As the plume given off during electrocauterisation can carry virus particles and friable bacterial spores, the use of high-frequency electrosurgical units in electrosectioning or desiccation modes should be used in conjunction with a smoke evacuator in which the viral or bacterial particles are taken up by charcoal filters. The collecting end of the smoke evacuator tubing should be no more than 2 cm from the surgical site or significant plume escape will occur.

7.4 Infrared coagulator

The infrared coagulator (Fig. 7.1) provides a relatively quick, cheap and effective treatment for blue/black tattoos and for certain cutaneous vascular lesions, including some vascular naevi, venous lakes and telangiectasia of Osler–Weber–Rendu syndrome, as well as for myxoid cysts. The infrared coagulator shares some of the properties of the neodymium:YAG laser;

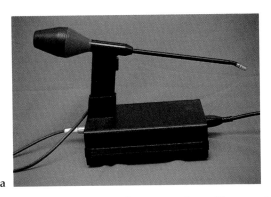
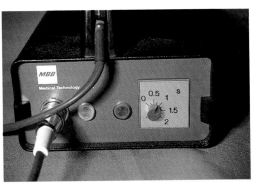

a   b

Fig. 7.1 Infrared coagulator. **a**. Device and **b**. control panel.

there is good penetration of the radiant energy and pulsing allows a predictable degree of thermal damage. It uses as its light source a tungsten halogen light bulb which emits light in the spectral band of 400–2700 nm, the emission being maximal at 900–960 nm. The energy emitted is in the form of non-coherent light which produces non-specific thermal skin injury. This radiation is reflected, by means of a gold-plated reflector, down a rigid quartz guide to a sapphire contact cap which allows radiant energy to be passed to the skin. An electronic timer sets the duration of each pulse between 0 and 1.5 s. The duration of the pulse has a direct relationship to the depth of tissue injury. Thermal damage in the surrounding tissue may lead to scar formation. The use of the infrared coagulator usually requires some form of local anaesthetic. During the treatment of tattoos there should be a slight spot to spot overlap until the area of the tattoo has been covered; it seems best to start with pulses of around 0.75 s increasing to about 1.25 s if necessary. For the treatment of vascular naevi, pulses of 0.4 s can induce clearance of the lesion with little change in the surrounding collagen. Recently, the infrared coagulator has been used to treat resistant viral warts. After anaesthesia is achieved, the wart is treated with overlapping pulses of 1.5–2.25 s, sufficient to induce blanching or opacification of the surface of the wart. Lesions treated in this way often develop haemorrhagic blisters which heal in 2–3 weeks. Large warts may be treated in sections.

7.5 Cautery

Cautery units rely on the heat generated in an electric wire, due to the resistance of an electric current passing through it, to cause heat destruction of tissues. A step-down transformer in the cautery box reduces the voltage to about 5 V and steps up the current to around 15 A. The heat controlled in the electrode tip can be varied using a rheostat dial on the cautery box. Available tips for the cautery include: (i) those suitable for tissue destruction and coagulation; (ii) a spade-like tip useful for snipping skin tags or polyps; and (iii) a pointed tip for the coagulation of small vascular lesions such as spider naevi. When tissue destruction is the main aim the cautery tip should be at a dull or cherry-red colour, when significant charring of tissue can be achieved. The advantages of electrocautery include its low cost, controllable tissue damage, useful for the destruction of tumours, and the fact that electrocautery works in a field containing blood, so that haemostasis is often easier to achieve than with other electrosurgical modalities. Another advantage of the electrocautery unit is that it can be used safely in patients with a pacemaker.

A disadvantage of cautery is that significant tissue charring can occur, making the healing process longer and can sometimes lead to a hypertrophic scar. However, with good technique both good cosmetic results and cure rates can be achieved for lesions such as basal cell carcinoma, especially in the elderly. Another disadvantage of cautery is the strong smell from cauterised tissue which may be disconcerting for the patient and disturbing for the user.

Cold point cautery

In the treatment of lesions such as spider naevi it is possible to use cold point cautery, in which a central fine cautery tip is heated by a surrounding coil of wire at its upper portion. This allows the cold point cautery tip to be heated in a more controlled fashion, thus enabling heat to be delivered to a small lesion in a precise way such that scarring is minimised.

Recently, small cordless cautery units have been developed which use rechargeable batteries. These are particularly useful for dermatologists who wish to use this treatment modality at several locations.

Bibliography

Adam JE. The technique of curettage surgery. *J Am Acad Dermatol* 1986; 15: 697–702.

Boughton RS, Spencer SK. Electrosurgical fundamentals. *J Am Acad Dermatol* 1987; 16: 862–7.

Colver GB, Jones RL, Cherry GW, Dawber RP, Ryan TJ. Precise dermal damage with an infrared coagulator. *Br J Dermatol* 1986; 114: 603–8.

Colver GB. The infra-red coagulator in dermatology. *Dermatol Clin* 1989; 7: 155–67.

Kemmett D, Colver GB. Myxoid cysts treated by infra-red coagulation. *Clin Exp Dermatol* 1994; 19: 118–20.

Kirkham P, Langtry JAA. Infrared coagulation of resistant viral warts. *Br J Dermatol* 1995; 133: 48S.

Sebben JE. The hazards of electrosurgery. *J Am Acad Dermatol* 1987; 16: 869–71.

Sebben JE. The status of electrosurgery in dermatological practice. *J Am Acad Dermatol* 1988; 19: 542–9.

Tromovitch TA, Glogau RG, Stegman SJ. The Shaw scalpel. *J Dermatol Surg Oncol* 1983; 9: 316–19.

8 Basic ellipse biopsy

It is important to decide whether one wishes to excise a lesion entirely for histopathology, as would be the case, for example, in a suspect naevus, or whether one wishes to make an incisional biopsy, in which only some of the lesion is excised. Inclusion of adjacent normal skin in an incisional biopsy makes it easier for the pathologist to assess the histopathological changes. In general, excisional biopsies should be carried out on discrete lesions, such as naevi, basal cell carcinomas or other solitary tumours, while incisional biopsies are more likely to be used for diagnostic purposes. Orientation of an incisional biopsy at right angles to the border of a lesion allows assessment of the change from pathological to normal tissue and also allows studies such as immunofluorescence and electron microscopy to be carried out on both lesional and non-lesional skin (Fig. 8.1). A further choice lies between an ellipse biopsy or punch biopsy. In general, pathologists prefer ellipse biopsies, since they provide more tissue allowing better assessment of the lesion in conjunction with the normal surrounding skin and yield satisfactory amounts of deeper tissue such as the subcutaneous fat. The latter is particularly important when considering a panniculitis. While punch biopsies can often reach subcutaneous fat, it is usually difficult to get good biopsy material from deep fat.

Punch biopsy techniques are none the less useful since they enable a histopathological diagnosis to be achieved while leaving only a small scar.

8.1 Design of the ellipse biopsy

Careful thought should be given to the design of the ellipse before performing any biopsy, with regard to the cosmetic result, the optimum tissue requirements for diagnosis or tumour clearance, and the nature of the ellipse itself. The size and orientation of the ellipse may to some extent be determined by the shape and position of the lesion to be excised, but extra care in planning should be taken around so-called free margins such as the ear rims, eyelids and lips which may be distorted by poorly designed scar orientation. Particularly important is the region around the lower eyelid since, if incorrect, biopsy design can lead to scarring with subsequent ectropion formation. Excisions from the lower eyelid are usually best performed with the long axis of the ellipse perpendicular to the free edge of the lower eye, such that contraction in wound healing will be at right angles to the free margin, and will not result in ectropion.

8.2 Relaxed skin tension lines

The best cosmetic results during skin surgery can be achieved by placing incision lines in, or parallel to, the so-called relaxed skin tension lines, which can be demonstrated by observation of the wrinkle lines and the effect of pinching the skin (see Chapter 3, Section 3.6). If the optimal orientation is still unclear the lesion can be excised as a circle in the first instance; after undermining the surrounding tissue, the wound will be pulled into a more oval shape, the long axis of which corresponds to the direction of the relaxed skin tension lines. The circular defect can then be fashioned into an ellipse or the resulting oval defect can be closed from the centre, with subsequent repair of the resulting 'dog-ears' at either end. This method may result in a shorter scar than would be achieved through more theoretical planning.

Having decided the direction in which the long axis of the ellipse should be placed, the ellipse should be drawn around the lesion before introducing the local anaesthetic, to prevent tissue distortion, which might make subsequent planning of the ellipse more difficult. Marking of the skin can be done either using a surgical skin marker, such as the Viomedex® skin marker (Fig. 8.2) which uses a non-toxic, blue-coloured dye. Alternatively, the area can simply be degreased using an alcohol swab and allowed to dry, when the planned excision is marked using a simple ball-point pen. One approach is to start by marking a circle around the lesion to be excised, and then making this the centre of the ellipse. The excision should have a length:width ratio of at least 3:1 and the apices should be at an angle of 30° (Fig. 8.3). After the area has been

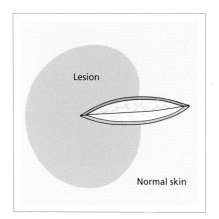

Fig. 8.1 Ellipse biopsy of skin lesion to include pathological and normal tissue.

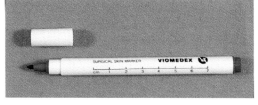

Fig. 8.2 Skin marker pen with centimetre ruler.

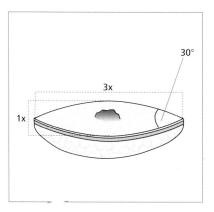

Fig. 8.3 The basic ellipse biopsy, with the length being three times that of the total width and angles at the apices of 30°.

marked the skin can then be anaesthetised by simple local infiltration around the site.

8.3 Incisional technique

Incisions are best carried out using a No. 15 scalpel blade with the scalpel held in the dominant hand and the index finger and thumb of the non-dominant hand placed on either side of the incision, thus keeping the skin under tension downward and away from the incising scalpel (Fig. 8.4). At the apex of the ellipse, the incision should be made using the point of the scalpel held in the vertical position, but as the incision progresses along the line of the ellipse the belly of the scalpel should be used to make the incision; the tip should be used again at the other end of the ellipse (Fig. 8.5). Effort should be made to avoid extending the incisions past the apices of the ellipse causing 'cross-hatching' (Fig. 8.6). The scalpel should be maintained perpendicular to the skin surface during the incision, thus avoiding bevelling skin edges (Fig. 8.7). An exception to this rule is in hairy areas, such as the eyebrows, where it is best to keep the incision parallel to the angle of the emerging hair, thus avoiding transection of hair follicles, and ensuring a better cosmetic result in terms of hair regrowth.

The incision should be through the full thickness of the skin including the upper subcutaneous fat in order to optimise the tissue specimen for histological diagnosis; if panniculitis is suspected the full thickness of the

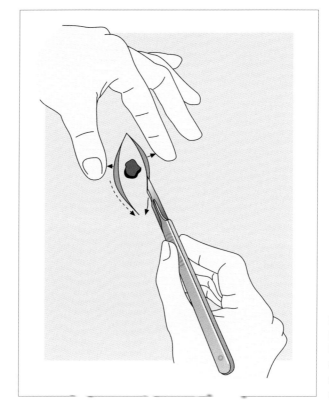

Fig. 8.4 Use of thumb and forefinger of non-dominant hand to steady skin while making incisions.

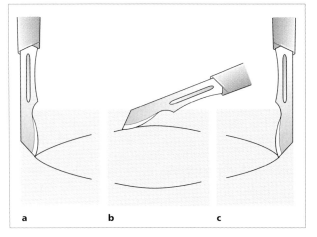

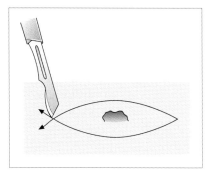

Fig. 8.6 Avoid cross-hatching by incising beyond apex of ellipse.

Fig. 8.5 a. Apex of ellipse cut with tip of blade held vertically; **b**. sides of ellipse cut with belly of blade; and **c**. end of ellipse cut with blade vertical.

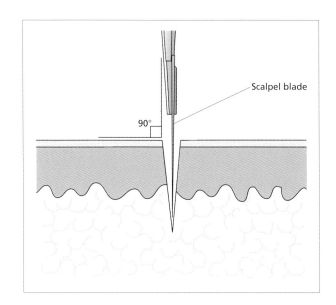

Fig. 8.7 Scalpel blade at right angles to skin surface throughout excision.

subcutaneous fat should be included. The depth of the excision will obviously be determined by the pathology of the lesion as well as by the location on the body. Once the skin incisions have been made on both sides of the ellipse, the tissue can be dissected free of the underlying fat. To avoid crush artefact to the skin being submitted for histopathology, it is best to catch the under surface of the tip of the apex using a skin hook, which can be used to pull the apex free of the wound, allowing a plane of dissection to be established for removal of the biopsy tissue (Fig. 8.8). Alternatively, toothed forceps can be used to hold the apex of the ellipse being removed if the pathology is located at the centre of the ellipse.

The ellipse can be dissected free using curved blunt-tipped dissection scissors (Steven's Tenotomy scissors, Cradle scissors or Metzenbaum scissors), making certain that the plane of dissection is the same throughout (Figs 8.9 & 8.10). There is a tendency for inexperienced operators to use a shallow plane of dissection at either end of the ellipse, and a deeper one in the centre, thus ending up with a bow-shaped excision specimen; when the skin is sutured this tends to leave a depression at the centre of the scar. When dissecting free the ellipse, the scissors should be placed in the wound with the tips parallel to the skin surface and advanced with the tips closed; the tips should only be opened during retraction of the scissors (see Fig. 8.9). This avoids the cutting of vital structures such as nerves and blood vessels during the process of freeing the ellipse.

An alternative approach has recently been described where the lesion is excised to create a circular defect and, after undermining in all directions, the optimum direction of closure is determined by suturing the centre of

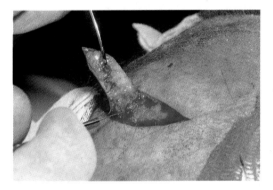

Fig. 8.8 Removal of specimen with skin hook.

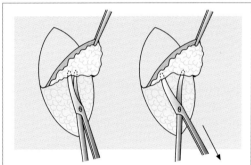

Fig. 8.9 Dissection of ellipse free from underlying tissue by blunt dissection.

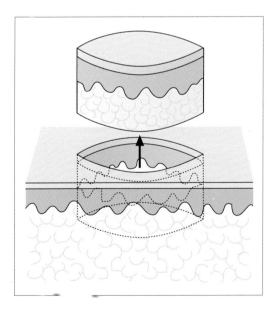

Fig. 8.10 Depth of ellipse at same level throughout its base.

the wound along lines of least resistance, which is usually parallel to relaxed skin tension lines. The resultant tissue mound at either end is then removed by a standard 'dog-ear' repair. This approach was found to result in significantly shorter scars and potentially better orientation of wounds than was achieved by simple ellipse excision. It was also noted that wounds on the trunk and limbs generally become more elliptical after excision, whereas the reverse tends to occur on the scalp and neck, where wounds often become more circular than a planned elliptical shape.

8.4 Undermining

For the most part, when performing ellipse excisions, the surgeon will be aiming to close the wound using direct side to side closure with the aid of sutures. However, in certain circumstances, this may not be necessary or desirable, and it may be possible to leave the wound open, and to let the wound heal over the next 4–6 weeks by secondary intention, dressing it daily with antibiotic ointments (see Chapter 13). This often leads to a very good cosmetic result and some skin surgeons prefer this approach on areas where scar tends to stretch, i.e. on the upper back and anterior chest.

Undermining of the surrounding skin is essential in order to achieve the best possible skin closure and to minimise tension on skin sutures. Subcutaneous sutures may then be placed, allowing the wound edges to be approximated, if necessary layer by layer to close dead space, such that the final superficial skin sutures are placed without any tension on wound edges. One potential disadvantage of undermining is that a space is created for blood accumulation, and thus more meticulous haemostasis is usually advisable.

Method of undermining

During undermining the skin edge should be elevated using a skin hook rather than forceps, which might crush the skin edge and compromise the final cosmetic result. Undermining is carried out using blunt-tipped scissors introduced with the tips closed and parallel to the skin surface (Fig. 8.11). Only when the scissors have been advanced to the desired degree should

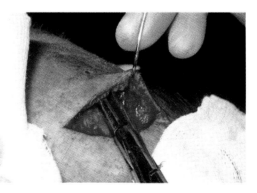

Fig. 8.11 Elevating skin surface with skin hook and undermining with a blunt-tipped instrument.

the scissors be opened to stretch the underlying tissue before being removed; the process is repeated until the desired skin mobility is achieved (Fig. 8.12). Such blunt dissection reduces the possibility of cutting vital structures including blood vessels and nerves. When a number of advancements of the scissors have been made, remaining tissue septa can be cut using the open blades of the scissors, but only under direct vision to avoid cutting vital structures.

Undermining is best carried out in the superficial fat in most areas, but in areas where the subcutaneous tissues are dense and thick, such as on the lower back, undermining at the level of deep subcutaneous tissue may be easier (Fig. 8.13). On the scalp, the subgaleal plane is usually the best area for undermining. On the face and neck, undermining in the superficial fat reduces the possibility of injury to nerves and blood vessels. Particular care in undermining should be taken around the temple and angle of jaw,

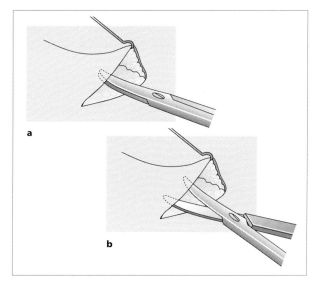

Fig. 8.12 a. Dissecting scissors advanced with blades closed and **b.** dissection with blades separated and withdrawn under direct vision.

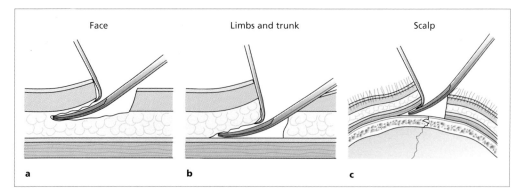

Fig. 8.13 Suggested levels for undermining on: **a.** the face in the superficial subcutaneous fat, **b.** on the limbs and trunk between the subcutaneous fat and fascia; and **c.** on the scalp below the galea.

where the temporal branch and mandibular branches of the facial nerve run superficially (see Chapter 3), but damage to these vital nerves can be avoided by dissection which remains within the level of the superficial fat.

The amount of undermining required will depend upon the tension on the wound and the size of the defect, and should be continued past the apices of the incision. Tension remaining in the wound can be assessed from time to time using two skin hooks to draw the edges of the wound together.

8.5 Haemostasis

During surgery, blood vessels will inevitably be cut, although bleeding may not be that excessive, especially when adrenaline has been used as a vaso-constrictor. One disadvantage of the use of adrenaline is that when its effects wear off, blood vessels may dilate, and bleeding may commence with consequent haematoma formation. Meticulous attention therefore should be paid to sealing off all blood vessels in the field to prevent post-operative bleeding. Large vessels may be encountered and should be clipped using artery forceps, followed by ligature of the vessel using an absorbable suture. It is preferable to use the needle of the suture to anchor the suture in the surrounding subcutaneous tissue before tying off the blood vessel. Other blood vessels can be sealed using bipolar electrosurgical electrodes or diathermy. All efforts should be made to keep these processes to a minimum to minimise tissue destruction and charring; factors that lead to higher post-operative infection rates. Chemical haemostats such as aluminium hydroxide or ferric sulphate (Monsel's solution) should be avoided as they are not likely to be sufficient for larger vessels, and they also decrease tissue viability which predisposes to wound infection. Insertion of a drain in large ellipse excisions to allow the externalisation of any blood or serous ooze occurring after wound closure is rarely necessary. After haemostasis has been achieved, all devitalised tissue and foreign material, including loose absorbable suture material, should be removed prior to wound closure.

8.6 'Dog-ear' repairs

Where the angle at the apices of an ellipse excision is greater than 30°, there will be a tendency for bunching up of excess tissue at either end of the wound closure, resulting in a 'dog-ear' (Fig. 8.14). It is sometimes possible to control the 'dog-ear' simply by placing sutures over it, especially in the

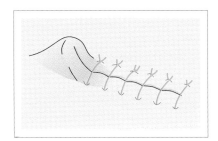

Fig. 8.14 'Dog-ear' at one end of closed wound.

elderly where the skin is quite forgiving. For 'dog-ears' that are larger or occur in younger people, a simple excision process can be carried out.

The apex of the 'dog-ear' is elevated using a skin hook or toothed forceps and pulled to one side such that the base of the 'dog-ear' lies in the same line of the wound (Fig. 8.15). The exposed side of the base is then cut with a scalpel. The triangular redundant skin is then pulled to the opposite side of the wound and a second incision is made along the line of the wound to the apex of the first incision (Fig. 8.16). This will remove the triangular excess of skin, allowing the wound to flatten down, and enabling it to be sutured in the normal way.

A comprehensive review of 'dog-ear' repairs and methods of suturing sides of unequal length is given in Chapter 20.

8.7 Wound closure and suturing

Details of sutures used for closing wounds and suturing techniques have already been given in Chapter 6 and will only be described briefly here.

Sutures are clearly important for wound closure, but since they can invoke foreign body reactions and provide tracts for infection they should be kept to a minimum. Buried sutures should be used to close dead space and also to approximate the dermal edges, thus removing tension from the wound. Closure of dead space is particularly important when large subcutaneous cavities have been created, such as following the removal of subcutaneous cysts, where the wound should be closed in layers.

Dermal buried sutures are particularly important on areas of the body overlying large muscle groups, for example on the upper trunk, as the forces of tension on the wound following suture removal can be great, leading to stretched scars and impaired cosmetic result. It is important to use the inverted knot buried suture when placing dermal sutures so that the knot is at the bottom of the incision, minimising the likelihood of the suture ends protruding from the wound or suture 'spits'. If there is some tension on the wound at the time of placing the subcutaneous sutures, it is useful to have

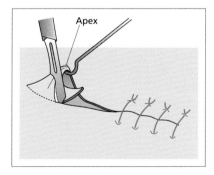

Fig. 8.15 Excess skin of 'dog-ear' pulled to one side using skin hook and incised to its apex in line with the original incision.

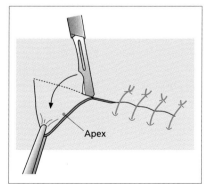

Fig. 8.16 The redundant tissue pulled to the opposite side of the wound using tissue forceps and incised to the apex along the direction of the initial incision.

an assistant push the edges of the wound together while the knot is being tied in place, since this results in better approximation of the wound sides. The strength of the suture material used will depend on the area where they are being placed: for areas such as the face or limbs, Vicryl® or Dexon® sutures are best, while on areas such as the upper trunk where greater skin support is required, polydioxanone sulphate (PDS® or Maxon®) sutures should be considered. The number of throws on buried sutures should be limited to two or three, and the tails cut short close to the knot to minimise tissue reaction. The sutures must be placed at the same level on either side of the incision to avoid causing an uneven wound edge, and although they should be placed in the upper dermis they should not be placed too near the epidermal surface, as this may cause suture extrusion in the weeks following wound closure. Following the placement of the subcutaneous sutures, the edges of the wound should be well approximated, not under tension, and ready for the skin sutures. Skin closure will most commonly be carried out using the simple interrupted skin suture technique, and the suture used will depend on the size and tension of the wound and the anatomical site: 5/0 or 6/0 synthetic (Prolene®, Ethilon®, Novafil®) sutures being used on the face, and 3/0 or 4/0 sutures being used on the trunk and back. The needle should be grasped by the suture holder about halfway along the needle, and the needle should enter at 90° to the skin, continue on this vertical path through the dermis, and only begin to curve after reaching the subcutaneous fat. This process is then reversed on needle exit. This will cause slight eversion of the wound edges, reducing the possibility of wound inversion and stretching. It may occasionally be advisable, or necessary, to exit the wound at its mid-point before completing the suture by reinserting the needle into deep subcutaneous tissue and passing vertically up through the skin surface of the opposite side of the wound. The suture is then tied using the square knot and the ends cut to a length of approximately 5 mm.

When closing the wound, it is probably best to use the method of halving. The first suture is placed in the centre of the ellipse, the second and third sutures are placed in the centres of the residual wound lengths and so forth until the wound is closed (Fig. 8.17). This method allows the equal distribution of tension along the wound edges and permits the 'sewing in' of wound edges, which may be slightly different in length.

Other suturing techniques that can be used for skin closure are discussed in greater detail in Chapter 6; in particular, the running continuous subcutaneous suture, which decreases the number of skin punctures on either side of the wound, considerably reduces the number of suture marks and

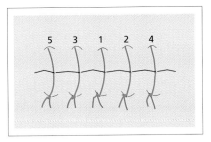

Fig. 8.17 Wound closed by the method of halving; sequence of suture placing in accordance with the numbers alongside sutures.

may result in a better cosmetic closure. However, if a wound haematoma or infection occurs, then the whole running subcutaneous suture has to be removed, whereas, if interrupted sutures have been used, removal of one or two sutures may be sufficient to allow drainage of the wound. For smaller ellipses newer closure materials can be considered, such as tissue glues (Histoacryl®); if there is little or no tension, skin closure tapes across the wound may be sufficient to keep the wound edges approximated. These latter methods may be particularly useful for wound closure in children.

8.8 Pathology

As soon as the biopsy is taken, it should immediately be placed in the correct fixative in a bottle labelled with the patient's name, date and site of the lesion. Thought should be given to selecting the fixatives to avoid an unnecessary second biopsy at a later stage. For routine histology 10% buffered formalin is a suitable fixative. If electron microscopy is being considered, part of the biopsy should be placed in Karnovsky's fixative, while for immunofluorescence the biopsy can either be snap frozen and placed in a small labelled plastic tube for immersion in liquid nitrogen, or placed in Michel's fixative for despatch to the laboratory. For other specialised investigations such as culture for bacteria, atypical mycobacterium and fungi, the relevant laboratories should be contacted to determine the most appropriate transport medium. It is essential when specimens are taken from more than one site that each biopsy is placed in a separate clearly labelled bottle. If the biopsy is particularly small, it can be placed on a piece of blotting paper with the epidermis upwards, so that it is correctly orientated when it arrives at the laboratory. It is also extremely important to fill in the histopathology request form fully to help the pathologist reach a correct diagnosis. In addition to the patient's name, age, identification number and sex, it should state whether the biopsy was intended to be a formal excision of a lesion or simply an incisional diagnostic biopsy. A clinical description with the site of the lesion and its duration, if known, should be given, with the clinician's suspected diagnosis. All skin biopsies taken should be sent for histological diagnosis, as sometimes even the most banal lesion turns out to be more sinister; even experienced clinicians will not always make a correct clinical diagnosis.

The specimen, together with the form, should then be packed in a self-sealing plastic bag and transported to the laboratory as soon as possible. Laboratory staff should be warned if the patient is known to suffer from a particular infectious disease (e.g. hepatitis), and the bag should be marked appropriately with a biohazard label. If transport involves postage, the bag must be packed in a suitable box surrounded by sufficient packing material to absorb the fixative fluid should the biopsy container be broken during the postage process. By adhering to these rules the best possible advice and service from the histopathological laboratory will be obtained.

Bibliography

Abide JM, Nahai F, Bennett RG. The meaning of surgical margins. *Plast Reconstr Surg* 1984; 73: 492–6.

Bart RS, Kopf AW. Techniques of biopsy of cutaneous neoplasms. *J Dermatol Surg Oncol* 1979; 5: 979–87.

Borges AF. Dog-ear repair. *Plast Reconstr Surg* 1982; 69: 707–13.

Davis TS, Graham WP, Miller SH. The circular excision. *Ann Plast Surg* 1980; 4: 21–4.

Dzubow LM. The dynamics of dog-ear formation and correction. *J Dermatol Surg Oncol* 1985; 11: 722–8.

Freeman RG. Handling of pathologic specimens for gross and microscopic examination in dermatologic surgery. *J Dermatol Surg Oncol* 1982; 8: 673–9.

Hudson-Peakcock MJ, Lawrence CM. Comparison of wound closure by means of dog-ear repair and elliptical excision. *J Am Acad Dermatol* 1995; 32: 627–30.

Larson PO. Review: topical hemostatic agents for dermatologic surgery. *J Dermatol Surg Oncol* 1988; 14: 623–34.

Robinson JK. *Fundamentals of Skin Biopsy*. Chicago: Year Book Medical Publishers, 1986.

Zitelli JA. Tips for a better ellipse. *J Am Acad Dermatol* 1990; 22: 101–3.

9 Punch biopsy

The punch biopsy method enables removal of a core of skin for biopsy using a relatively simple and quick technique. It has the advantage of maintaining tissue orientation and can even, for small lesions, be used to perform an excisional biopsy. However, it is more often used to perform incisional diagnostic biopsies of larger lesions, especially when it is desirable to leave only a small surgical scar, for example on the face. It has the disadvantage for the histopathologist of producing only a small biopsy specimen with little or no surrounding normal skin for comparison; an inexperienced operator may take too superficial a punch, preventing assessment of pathology in the subcutaneous fat.

9.1 Punches available

Most practitioners now use the widely available disposable, sterile punches which come in a range of sizes, including 2, 3, 4, 5, 6 and 8 mm diameter of circular cutting edge (Stiefel®, Fray Biopunch®), although reusable punches are available (the Keyes' punch). Recently, sterile disposable punches with an oval cutting edge, 3 × 7.5 mm and 4 × 8 mm have become available and will undoubtedly become more popular.

9.2 Technique of punch biopsy

Circular punch biopsy

After the skin has been cleaned with antiseptic and anaesthetised, the punch is held in the dominant hand between the thumb, middle and ring fingers with the index finger placed on the top of the punch head (Fig. 9.1). The skin surrounding the area to be biopsied should be placed under tension using the thumb and forefinger of the other hand to stretch the skin perpendicular to the relaxed skin tension lines, so that when the punch is removed the resulting wound will be oval or elliptical rather than round (Fig. 9.2). The biopsy is taken by placing the sharp, circular cutting edge on to the skin and exerting vertical downwards pressure on the punch while rotating the instrument (Fig. 9.3). This vertical pressure and circular motion is maintained until the cutting edge has reached the subcutaneous fat, at which stage the punch is withdrawn. This leaves a small core of tissue, held in place by the fat pedicle at its base, which can be lifted with a skin hook and snipped free of its base with scissors (Fig. 9.4). Forceps should not be used to grasp the tissue plug, as this is likely to produce tissue artefact. It is best to place the biopsy specimen on a piece of filter paper for a few minutes to dry before dropping it into the fixative solution; this helps the pathologist to properly orientate the tissue when it is received by the laboratory.

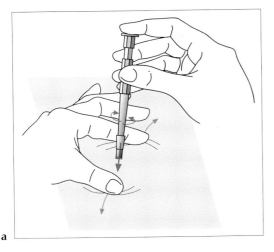

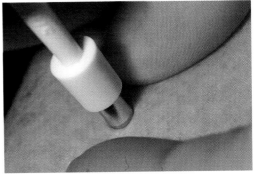

b

a

Fig. 9.1 a. Skin punch being rotated and pushed downward by the dominant hand while non-dominant hand stretches skin perpendicular to the relaxed skin tension lines. **b**. Circular punch being introduced to skin.

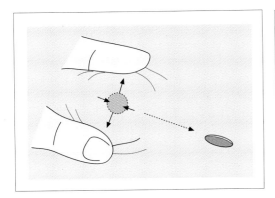

Fig. 9.2 Initially round defect created which, when fingers of non-dominant hand are released, becomes oval in shape.

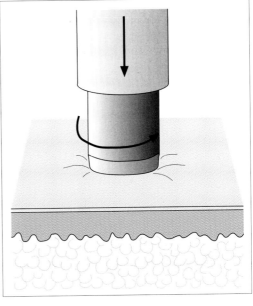

Fig. 9.3 The punch biopsy being taken by both rotational and vertical movements.

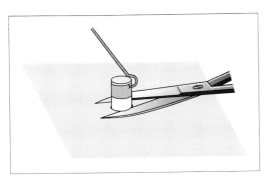

Fig. 9.4 Small skin plug being pulled up using a skin hook and snipped through the base with scissors.

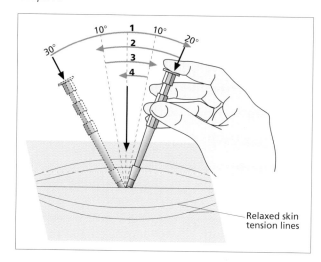

Fig. 9.5 Elliptical punch incising skin at 30° to the vertical, being rocked side to side with the dominant hand while vertical pressure is applied.

Bleeding from a punch biopsy site can usually be controlled by gentle pressure followed by suturing of the skin, but occasionally bleeding can be profuse if an artery has been cut by the punch. In this case, the bleeding vessel can usually be coagulated using either a hyfrecator or by cautery before the wound is sutured.

Some controversy exists as to whether the wound created by punch biopsy requires suturing. While reasonable cosmetic results can be achieved by leaving the wound to heal by granulation, the authors feel that it is best to use sutures to close the wound, especially for the larger punch sizes. The vertical mattress suture is often very useful for approximating both the deep dermis and the skin edge.

Elliptical punch biopsy

The technique for an elliptical punch biopsy is a slight modification of the above. Following placement of the punch directly over the lesion, initial cutting pressure to puncture the skin is applied with the punch tilted 30° off vertical at one of the proposed apices of the ellipse. The handle is then tilted back through the vertical and a similar puncture is made at the opposite proposed apex. Gentle rocking back and forth between 10° of the vertical while exerting downward pressure enables the incision to be made to the required depth (Fig. 9.5).

Bibliography

Eisen D. The oral mucosal punch biopsy. *Arch Dermatol* 1992; 128: 815–17.

10 Curettage and cautery

Two main forms of dermal curette are used in dermatological practice. The most common form in the UK is the cup-shaped curette which comes in a variety of sizes, while in the USA the open-headed fenestrated curette seems to be more popular. Dermal curettes have the property of being sharp enough to remove superficial soft lesions from the skin, but not be so sharp as to cut into the surrounding firmer, normal dermis. This property allows superficial lesions such as warts to be 'shelled out' of the skin with the minimum of dermal damage, thus leaving a good cosmetic result.

10.1 Indications for curettage

Curettage is most useful in small, superficial skin lesions with a soft texture which clearly separates them from the surrounding dermis. Such lesions include seborrhoeic keratoses, actinic keratoses, viral warts and superficial types of basal cell carcinoma and squamous cell carcinoma. It is not indicated for lesions with a strong fibrous tissue component, such as morphoeic-type basal cell carcinomas, where it is difficult to achieve a cleavage plane between the malignant lesion and the surrounding dermis.

10.2 Technique of curettage and cautery

Because the wound created by curettage is superficial it is usually adequate for the operator to use non-sterile procedure gloves during curettage and cautery. The skin is cleaned with a topical antiseptic and the skin beneath and around the lesion is injected with local anaesthetic. For very superficial lesions such as molluscum contagiosum, it may be possible to omit the anaesthetic injection as this may be more painful than the procedure.

During the procedure it is useful to stretch and stabilise the skin surrounding the lesion using the tips of the thumb and index finger placed on opposite sides of the lesion (Fig. 10.1). The curette is held between the thumb and index finger of the dominant hand and is drawn through the lesion with a steady yet firm downward scooping motion (Fig. 10.2a,b,c). Haemostasis can be achieved by cautery (Fig. 10.2c).

It is recommended that the bulk of the lesion be removed with a large curette, with smaller residual fragments being removed using a smaller sized curette; this is particularly important when dealing with a malignant lesion. For some lesions such as seborrhoeic warts, it may be advantageous to coagulate the lesion first by cautery or using a hyfrecator, thereby softening the tissue and permitting a better plain of cleavage to be achieved. When removing softer lesions such as basal cell carcinomas, one can usually feel a distinct difference between the firm normal skin and the softer tumour tissue, enabling the operator to assess when the lesion has been adequately removed.

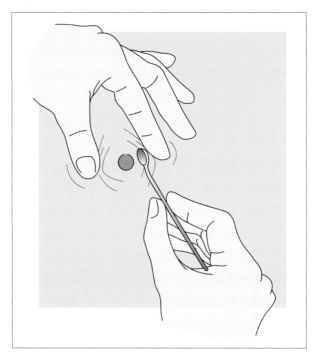

Fig. 10.1 Skin surrounding lesion held tense between the thumb and forefinger of the non-dominant hand, while lesion is curetted with spoon curette held in the dominant hand.

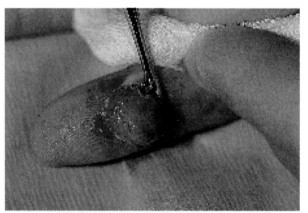

a

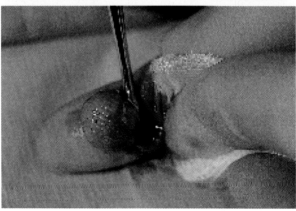

b

Fig. 10.2 a. Curette being introduced under the lesion; **b**. lesion being lifted by curette from skin.

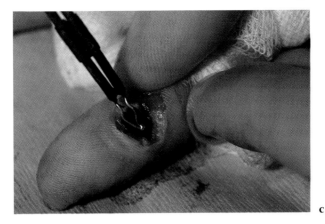

Fig. 10.2 *Continued*. **c**. Cautery being applied to defect created, for haemostasis.

c

For malignant tumours, it is prudent to cauterise the curetted area extensively, and to then repeat the curettage–cautery cycle three times until all suspected malignant tissue has been removed. It is also best to remove 2–5 mm of surrounding normal skin in an attempt to clear the marginal region of any microscopic finger-like projections of tumour. Cure rates for malignant tumours by curettage and cautery have been shown to be related to operator experience, but for basal cell carcinomas cure rates approach 95% if correctly performed.

10.3 Haemostasis

Haemostasis following curettage can be achieved using either cautery or hyfrecation to seal the blood vessels. A gauze pad is pressed over the wound, and as the gauze is partially pulled away the exposed area of the curetted wound can be coagulated. Cautery should not be overzealous, especially on areas such as the dorsa of hands where underlying nerves or tendons could be damaged. In the case of a malignant lesion, more extensive and repeated cautery may be desirable. For more superficial benign lesions such as molluscum contagiosum or seborrhoeic warts, a saturated solution of aluminium chloride hexahydrate (Driclor®, Anhydrol Forte®) can be used as a haemostat. Bleeding can initially be controlled by keeping the skin under tension between the thumb and forefinger, while the aluminium chloride hexahydrate solution is applied to the area using a cotton bud applicator. This seals superficial vessels, has the advantage of not leaving a charred surface and also reduces the possibility of scarring. Any late bleeding can usually be controlled by the application of gentle pressure using sterile gauze for about 5 min. Curettage and cautery can often be carried out in patients on anti-coagulants, provided the lesion is not deep and meticulous care is taken to achieve haemostasis during the procedure.

10.4 Wound care

Following haemostasis the wound can either be left exposed or covered with a simple dressing, under which a topical antibiotic ointment may be applied. The lesion will then form a crust over the course of 1 week to 10 days, which will eventually separate to leave a clean superficial granulating wound. It is rare for infection to be a problem following curettage and cautery, but pain, swelling or surrounding erythema may herald infection requiring systemic antibiotic therapy.

Occasionally, wounds, particularly of the forehead or temple, may heal with excessive granulation tissue. This can be treated by weekly application of a silver nitrate pencil, or if necessary by repeat light curettage.

Clearly, following removal of deep-seated lesions such as basal cell carcinomas some scarring, often depressed or hypopigmented, can occur. It is, in fact, unusual for a patient to be dissatisfied with the final cosmetic result.

10.5 Recurrence of tumour following curettage

In experienced hands the technique of curettage can achieve a 5-year cure rate in excess of 95%. Studies have shown it to be a simple, efficacious and cost-effective way of treating basal cell carcinomas; recurrences appear to be highest with less skilled operators. Patients treated in this way should be followed up for signs of recurrence, which is most likely to occur at the periphery of the treated area, for up to 5 years. Most recurrent basal cell carcinomas appear in the first 3 years following the procedure.

10.6 Histopathology

The tissue material that has been curetted off should be sent to the histopathologist for confirmation of the clinical diagnosis. However, curettage has the obvious disadvantage of not enabling the pathologist to assess whether or not the lesion has been adequately removed.

Bibliography

Adam JE. The technique of curettage surgery. *J Am Acad Dermatol* 1986; 15: 697–702.

Albright SD. Treatment of skin cancer using multiple modalities. *J Am Acad Dermatol* 1982; 7: 143–71.

Kopf A, Bart R, Schrager D, Lazar M, Popkin GL. Curettage–electrodesiccation treatment of basal cell carcinomas. *Arch Dermatol* 1977; 113: 439–43.

Sakura C, Calamel P. Comparison of treatment modalities for recurrent basal cell carcinoma. *Plast Reconstr Surg* 1979; 63: 492–6.

Salasche SJ. Curettage and electrodesiccation in the treatment of midfacial basal cell epithelioma. *J Am Acad Dermatol* 1983; 8: 496–503.

Silverman MK, Kopf AW, Grin CM, Bart RS, Levenstein MJ. Recurrence rates of treated basal cell carcinomas. Part 2: Curettage–electrodesiccation. *J Dermatol Surg Oncol* 1991; 17: 720–6.

Spiller WF, Spiller RF. Treatment of basal cell epithelioma by curettage and electrodesiccation. *J Am Acad Dermatol* 1984; 11: 808–14.

11 Shave biopsy

11.1 Indications and limitations

The shave biopsy method is a technique that allows the biopsy and flattening of elevated lesions on the skin with minimal dermal damage, thus usually achieving an excellent cosmetic result. It is perhaps one of the simplest procedures carried out in dermatological surgery and is probably most useful for 'flattening' intradermal naevi, especially around the facial area. It can be used to treat a wide range of other elevated skin lesions, including pyogenic granulomas, seborrhoeic keratoses, skin polyps, Bowen's disease and various benign adnexal skin tumours. On occasion it can be used to obtain tissue for histological confirmation of lesions such as basal cell carcinomas, prior to more definitive excisional surgery. Shave biopsy is not indicated where a full thickness biopsy or total excision of the lesion is required and certainly should not be carried out on potential melanoma lesions as this will make it impossible for the pathologist to assess the maximum thickness of the lesion.

11.2 Methods

The skin should be cleansed with a topical antiseptic; because the risk of infection is small, sterile gloves are not essential. The mode of delivery of the local anaesthetic should be carefully considered before proceeding with a shave biopsy. It is probably best to place the local anaesthetic around or deep to the lesion to be removed, rather than immediately under it; the latter will elevate the lesion. If this is not taken into account during the shave procedure, a small depression may result after the anaesthetic has been resorbed. If it is felt necessary to elevate the lesion by injecting local anaesthetic under it, this effect should be minimised by massaging the area to disperse the anaesthetic agent. Alternatively, it may be possible to shave the lesion such that the central portion is slightly elevated, to ensure that the lesion will be flat when the anaesthetic agent is resorbed.

During the procedure the skin surrounding the lesion is immobilised by placing it on stretch between the thumb and index finger. The lesion is then shaved parallel to the skin, usually with a No. 10 blade and scalpel; a No. 15 blade may be used for smaller lesions. Some dermatological surgeons prefer to use a single-edged razor blade, such as the Gillette Super Blue Blade®, as they feel that these are easier to control and offer a degree of flexibility not afforded by the scalpel blade.

The shaving technique is carried out using a to-and-fro movement of the scalpel blade held parallel to the skin surface (Figs 11.1 & 11.2). It is essential that this movement is kept in the same plane as the blade advances steadily, to prevent ragged excision. It is probably best to shave round the total circumference of the lesion first before finally shaving through the

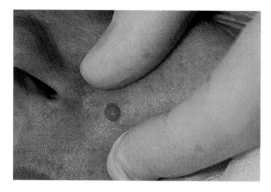

Fig. 11.1 Skin surrounding lesion being stabilised and stretched between the thumb and forefinger of the non-dominant hand.

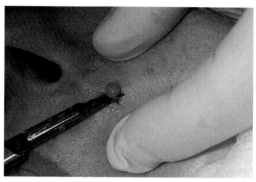

Fig. 11.2 Shave being initiated with scalpel blade parallel to skin surface.

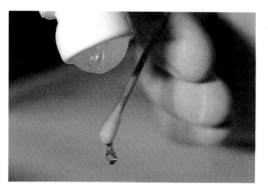

Fig. 11.3 Aluminium chloride hexahydrate solution released from container onto cotton bud.

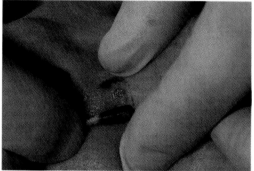

Fig. 11.4 Bud saturated with aluminium chloride hexahydrate being rubbed across shaved area while tension in skin is maintained between thumb and forefinger of the non-dominant hand to control bleeding.

central portion, removing it from the skin. The depth of the excision is also important. For many lesions it is best to aim for a shallow removal, which may result in only partial excision, as deeper shaves will result in a depression and more scarring. The small shaved specimen can be taken onto the scalpel blade and placed on a piece of tissue paper with the cut section down to dry for a few minutes before placing it in the fixative; this is to help the pathologist orientate the tissue fragment. Bleeding following shave biopsy is usually minimal and is probably best controlled by the topical use of saturated aluminium chloride hexahydrate solution (Driclor®, Anhydrol Forte®) squeezed onto a sterile cotton bud (Fig. 11.3), which is then rolled onto the cut surface of the skin (Fig. 11.4). Active bleeding during this procedure is minimised by tension placed on the wound by the thumb and forefinger of the operator. Alternatively, light cautery or hyfrecation can be applied, although these cause more tissue injury, and must be used judiciously if scarring is to be avoided.

11.3 Postoperative care

Because the wound created does not involve the full thickness of the dermis, infection and scarring are rare and the cosmetic result is usually excellent. However, when a naevus has been removed in this way it is possible that it may recur, or pigmentation may occur in the scar overlying the wound; the patient should be warned of this before the operative procedure. The wound itself can be left open, or if preferred, covered for the first day or so with a small Elastoplast® dressing under which the operator may wish to use an antibiotic ointment. The authors generally leave the wound open, thereafter instructing the patient to keep the area clean and dry for around 3 days. The area has normally re-epithelialised within 10 days.

Although less common than with excisional surgery, hypertrophic or keloidal scarring can occur following shave biopsy, especially on the upper chest and deltoid areas. Hypo- or hyperpigmentation may occur, especially in pigmented skins, and patients must be warned that terminal hairs almost certainly will not be removed, as the hair follicles usually lie deeper than the level of a satisfactory shave. Such terminal hairs may be removed later by epilation or electrolysis if desired.

Bibliography

Grabski WJ, Salasche SJ, Mulveney MJ. Razor-blade surgery. *J Dermatol Surg Oncol* 1990; 16: 1121–6.

12 Cryosurgery

Cryosurgery has been defined as the deliberate destruction of tissue by cold, in a controlled manner, and was probably first used in the 19th century when suitable refrigerants were becoming available. The original cryogens were carbon dioxide snow and liquid air, but these have now been superseded by liquid nitrogen, which has a boiling point of $-196°C$.

12.1 Physiology of cryosurgery

There has been considerable research on the various mechanisms by which cold can irreparably damage tissue cells. It was initially thought that ice crystals formed'would cause mechanical damage to cell membranes and disrupt cellular function. Although ice formation does occur during slow freezing, it is not, in itself, sufficient to kill cells.

The greatest damage to cells seems to be caused by the formation of intracellular ice when freezing is rapid. Repeated freeze–thaw cycles maximise this destructive effect, with electron microscopic studies on skin showing the destruction of all cell structures after two freeze–thaw cycles. The slow thaw after cryosurgery is most responsible for the tissue destruction as cell organelles such as mitochondria and endoplasmic reticulum are probably destroyed during the recrystallisation of ice. Other changes that bring about cell damage include: (i) disruption of the phospholipids in cell membranes; (ii) the creation of osmotic gradients when extracellular ice formation occurs; and (iii) ischaemia induced by vascular spasm during the freezing part of the cycle. Subsequent damage may also be caused by an immune reaction against antigens released following cryosurgery to tumour masses.

Tissue destruction by cryosurgery is not uniform and it is important to realise that some tissues are more resistant to damage than others. For example, it is known that melanocytes are very sensitive to the effects of cold damage, as are many tumour cells, whereas the connective tissue components, including dermal collagen and fibroblasts, seem to be relatively resistant to cold damage. Similarly, cartilage, unless infiltrated by tumour, is relatively resistant to cryosurgery. Cryosurgery damage to nerves can certainly give rise to local anaesthesia, but such sensory loss usually recovers over 18 months, even following prolonged freezing used for tumour eradication. It is also very important for clinicians to realise that viruses and bacteria are relatively resistant to low temperatures and that, indeed, viruses can be stored in liquid nitrogen. It is therefore not safe to presume that ulcerated lesions, which may be infected, will be eradicated of bacterial infection following cryosurgery. Viruses may potentially be transmitted through liquid nitrogen, especially when using a cotton bud or probe techniques.

12.2 Indications

Cryosurgery has been used to treat a wide variety of non-malignant and malignant skin lesions as shown in Table 12.1.

Lentigo maligna can be successfully treated by cryosurgery although this is more controversial, with many now believing that such lesions are best excised to reduce recurrence rates and to avoid missing an early lentigo maligna melanoma which may not be apparent except on histopathology (see Chapter 17).

12.3 Liquid nitrogen storage

Of all the cryogens, liquid nitrogen is the most readily available, and the most widely used. It has the advantage of being inexpensive, but must be stored after delivery in a Dewar® flask from which it will slowly evaporate. Dewar® flasks range in size from 5 to 50 L and have a static holding time ranging from 6 to 122 days, respectively. Liquid nitrogen can then be transferred from the Dewar® flask to a liquid nitrogen flask or cryogun by means of either a tipping stand or a withdrawal pump, which delivers up to 8 L of liquid nitrogen per minute. Whichever withdrawal method is used, it is advisable to wear a visor and also protective gloves in case of splashes. Adequate ventilation should also be available to prevent the build up of nitrogen levels in the work atmosphere. Liquid nitrogen can be readily obtained directly from an oxygen supplier (British Oxygen in the UK); alternatively, office practitioners may find it cheaper and more convenient to arrange a supply from a local hospital.

12.4 Contact techniques

Cotton buds

Cryotherapy may be delivered to a lesion by means of a cotton bud wound onto the end of an orange stick dipped into the liquid nitrogen container, such as a rigid polystyrene or metal cup, and then held against the skin. The depth of freeze induced by such a method is limited, and this technique certainly cannot be used for the eradication of tumours. The technique is, however, suitable for more superficial lesions including viral warts, actinic keratoses and molluscum contagiosum lesions. It is also often much less frightening for children when a cotton bud is used. It is essential that the bud tip be smaller than the lesion being treated so that one can observe the spread of ice throughout the lesion. The bud should be held vertically on the lesion, as opposed to being at an angle which often leads to excessive blistering in surrounding skin (Fig. 12.1). For the treatment of a superficial lesion, such as a viral wart, the aim is to produce ice formation extending beyond the lesion itself to include a rim of normal tissue of about 1 mm.

When treating infected lesions such as viral warts, it is important that the cotton bud does not contaminate a container which may subsequently be used in the treatment of another patient. The use of the cotton bud method has a lot to commend it: it is cheap, requires little capital expense, is easy to use and can often be performed by nurse practitioners.

Table 12.1 The treatment of skin lesions by cryosurgery.

Condition	Freeze–thaw time (s)	Lateral freeze (mm)
Warts		
Plane	1 × 5	None
Common	1 × 10	1
Plantar	1 × 10	1
Filiform	1 × 5	1
Mosaic	2 × 20	2
Molluscum contagiosum	To ice formation only	None
Seborrhoeic warts	1 × 10	1–2
Solar keratoses	1 × 10	1
Bowen's disease (including erythroplasia of Queyrat)	1 × 20–30	1–2
Pyogenic granuloma	1 × 15	1
Spider naevi	1 × 15	None
Orf	2 × 10	3
Cysts		
Epidermoid	1 × 15	
Digital synovial	1 × 30	Punctured cyst, 2–3
Oral mucous	1 × 10–20	
Keloids	1 × 30	1–2
Dermatofibromas	1 × 30	2–3
Rhinophyma	1 × 20	
Tattoos (amateur)	1 × 30	
Acne cysts	1 × 10	
Venous lakes	1 × 15–25	Cryoprobe recommended
Ingrowing toenails (granulation tissue)	1 × 20–30	
Tumours		
Keratoacanthoma	2 × 30	5
Lymphocytoma cutis	1 × 15–20	2–3
Basal cell carcinoma	2 × 30	2–3
Squamous cell carcinoma	2 × 30	2–3
Lentigo maligna	2 × 30	5 (excision recommended)
Kaposi's sarcoma	2 × 10–20 (macular)	3
	2 × 30–60 (papular)	3

For small skin lesions such as skin tags, a modification of this method can be used. Large metal non-toothed forceps can be dipped into liquid nitrogen for around 30 s before grasping the stalk of the skin tag for some 10 s (Fig. 12.2a,b). Skin tags frozen in this way will usually separate within 10 days.

Aerosol cryotherapy

This technique has gained popularity, especially among general practitioners, because of its convenience, although liquid nitrogen is a much cheaper option after the initial investment in equipment. Because of the

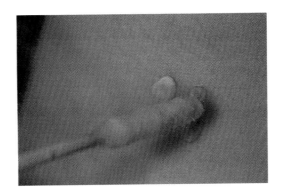

Fig. 12.1 Lesion being treated with liquid nitrogen by application of cotton bud.

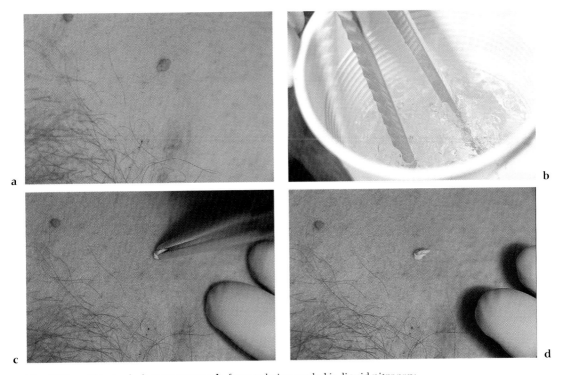

a

b

c

d

Fig. 12.2 a. Skin tag before treatment; **b**. forceps being cooled in liquid nitrogen; **c**. skin tag being held with cold forceps; and **d**. resultant frozen skin tag.

size of the cotton bud applicator, it is less accurate and more difficult to use than an ordinary cotton bud.

One such aerosol is the Histofreezer® which utilises dimethylether propane to provide a convenient way of delivering cryotherapy when liquid nitrogen is not available. The spray is delivered to the cotton bud by means of a hollow tube and its evaporation can achieve skin cooling to −50°C. It is not suitable for the treatment of neoplastic lesions.

Another aerosol device for cryosurgery, the Verruca-Freeze®, which utilises chlorodifluoromethane as the cryogen, has recently become available. The device is used in conjunction with cones of varying size which limit the spread of the spray from a narrow exhaust tube.

12.5 Spray technique

The use of the hand-held cryogun, which operates under a working pressure of approximately 6 psi, is the mainstay of cryotherapy. The larger standard gun (Cryogun® 2) has a holding time of up to 24 h, and the smaller Cryogun® mini (Fig. 12.3), which is about one-third smaller, has a holding time of about 12 h. Cryoguns come with nozzle attachments with apertures of varying diameter for spray delivery (Fig. 12.4); the A size nozzle delivers the largest spray and the D size nozzle the smallest spray for delicate work. For delivering liquid nitrogen to a defined area, neoprene cones, which vary in diameter from 5 to 38 mm, are available; they are useful for restricting the area of freezing (Fig. 12.5).

Standard auroscope earpieces can be used if neoprene cones are not available, or for the treatment of very small skin lesions (Fig. 12.6). Similarly, adhesive putty or Plasticene® can be used to make a small mould to apply around an area to be treated. It is possible to move the lower lid

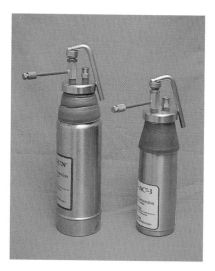

Fig. 12.3 Cry-ac® spray 2 and mini Cry-ac® spray gun.

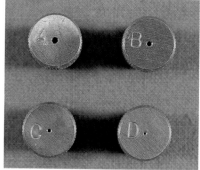

Fig. 12.4 Nozzles suitable for cryosurgery ranging from A (largest) to D (smallest).

away from the globe of the eye during cryosurgery to the lid using a plastic spoon, thus protecting the cornea and conjunctiva. Other accessories include an extension spray for use in cavities such as the mouth, and cryo-probe attachments, which are particularly useful for cryosurgery on mucous membranes (Fig. 12.7). Cryoprobes come in a number of different configurations and sizes with flat, rounded and pointed application surfaces. If used on skin, a thin layer of lubricant jelly should be applied to the skin to ensure the probe will adhere to the skin after some 5–6 s. After freezing has been completed, the probe will remain adherent to mucosa or skin for 10–30 s until thawing allows separation of the probe from the ice-ball. Sterilisation of cryoprobe tips should be carried out before their reuse to prevent any possibility of cross-infection between patients.

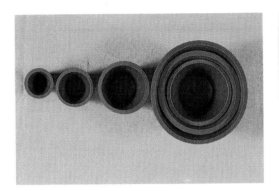

Fig. 12.5 Neoprene cones used for restricting areas of freeze.

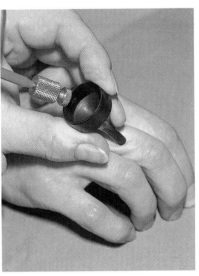

Fig. 12.6 Auroscope used to deliver liquid nitrogen spray to small lesion.

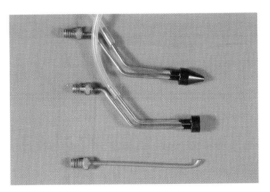

Fig. 12.7 Attachments for Cry-ac® spray. Conical-shaped (top), flat-bottomed probe (middle) and elongated spray gun (bottom).

12.6 Cryosurgery for benign and pre-malignant conditions

Cryosurgery compares favourably with other forms of treatment and has the advantages of not requiring anaesthetic, being mobile and able to be used on a wide variety of patients, even those with poor general health.

12.7 General cryosurgery

For benign and pre-malignant conditions of the skin, usually one single cycle of freeze–thaw is sufficient, and the length of the freeze–thaw cycle is indicated in Table 12.1. These times are given as general guidance but each patient should be treated individually according to thickness, size, location and character of the lesion being treated. Spray techniques give a much more rapid skin freeze than either cotton bud or cryoprobe techniques.

The freeze–thaw cycle is a vitally important concept central to the practice of cryosurgery. During this cycle, the area is frozen by the spray until the area that is to be treated is uniformly white and the area of ice formation has extended 2–3 mm beyond the margin of the area to be treated. At this stage counting begins, thus determining the freeze–thaw cycle in seconds. The liquid nitrogen applicator is then used to maintain this iceball without letting it expand or decrease in size for the required length of time, as suggested (Figs 12.8 & 12.9). After this time the application of cryogen is stopped and the tissue allowed to completely thaw.

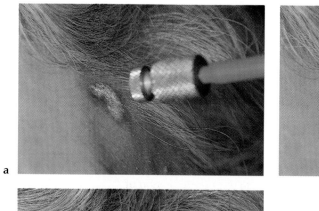

a

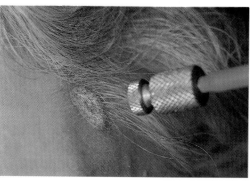

b

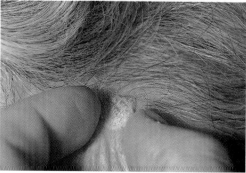

c

Fig. 12.8 a. Ice formation in lesion. **b**. Lesion frozen, together with rim of normal tissue. **c**. Assessing degree of iceball between thumb and forefinger.

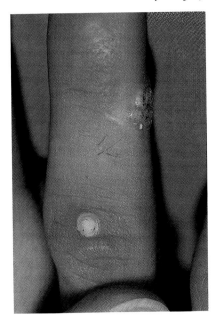

Fig. 12.9 Lesion treated with 1–2 mm
of ice formation on normal skin.

12.8 Cryosurgery in the treatment of skin cancer

Cryosurgery can be used to treat superficial, nodular or ulcerated basal cell carcinomas, and squamous cell carcinomas that have developed within an actinic keratosis. It is not suitable for tumours that have ill-defined borders such as morphoeic basal cell carcinomas. It is usually best reserved for tumours that are less than 2 cm in diameter. Cryosurgery can also be used for tumours overlying cartilage and bone, as these tissues are relatively resistant to cryo-injury and chondronecrosis is unusual, except if the cartilage is invaded by tumour. It is useful in circumstances that preclude excisional surgery, such as poor health, difficulty in attending a hospital-based clinic or the treatment of multiple tumours at one visit. Cryosurgery has been used successfully for the treatment of Kaposi's sarcoma in patients with acquired immune deficiency syndrome (AIDS) and also for malignant melanoma, but it is not recommended as a standard treatment for melanoma.

It is clearly essential that cell death occur in all areas where the tumour exists. It is advisable to mark a 5 mm margin outside the visible margin of the tumour, and the line of ice formation should be brought to at least this margin. Cryosurgery for eradication of tumours does not require the use of a thermocouple for temperature monitoring, provided the basic principles are understood and proper technique is adhered to; local anaesthesia is usually not required. The initial freezing can either be by the open spray, through a cone or by using a cryoprobe. A common way of delivering the cryogen is by open spray or by directing the spray into a neoprene cone placed over the tumour. Freezing is more rapid using a cone spray technique, and a greater depth of ice formation is achieved than with the open spray or probe methods. The cryoprobe method is useful for the treatment of lesions on mucosal surfaces, and has the advantage of a more predictable area and depth of tissue freezing. The main disadvantage of the probe relates to the necessity to avoid movement, as loss of probe adherence will interfere with the heat exchange and result in inadequate freezing.

Whichever method is chosen it is essential to use at least two freeze–thaw cycles for eradication of tumour cells. After the initial freezing, which will usually be for 30 s, the tumour site should be allowed to rewarm slowly as this is the time when most tissue destruction will occur. Time for total thawing should be at least three times the length of time taken for the freeze, after which a second freeze–thaw cycle is undertaken.

Following such long freeze–thaw cycles there will be a lot of tissue reaction with oedema and blistering. To minimise these reactions, potent topical corticosteroids such as clobetasol ointment (Dermovate®) may be applied, and a non-steroidal anti-inflammatory drug prescribed, which may also decrease tissue inflammation. There are some sites that do particularly well with cryosurgery: these include the external ear, the upper surfaces of the nose and the lower eyelid, whereas it is relatively contra-indicated on the lower legs where healing is slow and secondary infection can occur. Skin cancers treated in accordance with the above instructions have an overall cure rate of over 90% and often resolve with minimal scarring.

12.9 Cryosurgery in HIV patients

Cryosurgery may be a relatively risk-free treatment, compared to other forms of surgery, of some skin conditions in HIV-positive patients. Cryosurgery can be used for molluscum contagiosum, warts and condylomata accuminata using the spray technique. Kaposi's sarcoma also responds well to cryosurgery, especially in the case of thin lesions less than 1 cm in diameter. Treatment can be undertaken with freeze–thaw cycles of 30 s, but for large and deeper lesions longer freeze–thaw cycles may be associated with a poor cosmetic result and radiotherapy may be superior. If cryoprobes or neoprene cones come in contact with the patient they must be autoclaved following the procedure. Similarly, if liquid nitrogen spray is used to treat an ulcerated lesion, blood may be splattered onto the tip and, therefore, cryosurgery spray tips should also be autoclaved between patients.

12.10 Complications of cryosurgery

It is absolutely essential that patients be warned of the expected outcome of their treatment if complaints are to be avoided. All patients must be warned before treatment is initiated to expect blistering (Fig. 12.10), tissue swelling and pain. Occasionally, a patient may experience a vasovagal attack during or shortly after the procedure. Blistering increases where the radius of freezing has extended well beyond the margins of the lesion (Fig. 12.11a,b). Patients should be instructed to puncture blisters using a sterile needle (Fig. 12.11c) and to apply an antiseptic cream to prevent infection. Patients should receive instruction regarding pain management; unless contra-indicated, aspirin or paracetamol can be suggested. Instructions are

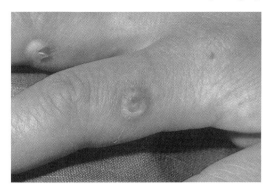

Fig. 12.10 Blistering that may result following cryosurgery. (Courtesy of Dr E.A. Bingham, Royal Victoria Hospital, Belfast.)

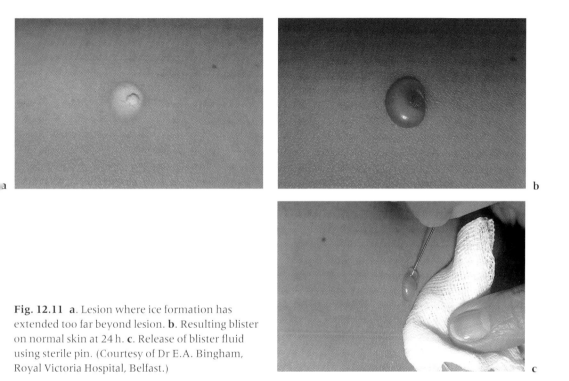

Fig. 12.11 a. Lesion where ice formation has extended too far beyond lesion. **b**. Resulting blister on normal skin at 24 h. **c**. Release of blister fluid using sterile pin. (Courtesy of Dr E.A. Bingham, Royal Victoria Hospital, Belfast.)

probably best given in the form of a handout with a contact telephone number in the event of problems developing.

The degree of oedema following cryosurgery is often difficult to predict, idiosyncratic and maximum in soft tissue sites such as peri-orbitally, the labia minora or foreskin; it is greatest in the elderly. Occasionally, it is so severe as to cause tense haemorrhagic blisters (Fig. 12.12). Bleeding can occur with aggressive anti-tumour doses of cryotherapy and this may be delayed for up to 14 days resulting from tissue necrosis within a tumour.

It is not uncommon for some degree of sensory impairment to occur following prolonged tissue freezes, but sensory recovery usually takes place. Atrophic scarring can occur with prolonged freeze–thaw cycles.

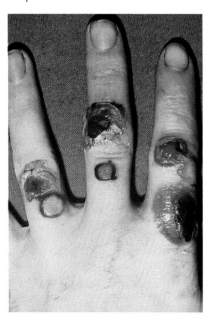

Fig. 12.12 Haemorrhagic blisters following excessive liquid nitrogen application.

Hypertrophic scarring is uncommon following cryotherapy and indeed cryotherapy can be used to treat such scars (see Chapter 21). Pigmentary changes are, however, much more common, even in white skin; hypopigmentation being common and often permanent, although post-inflammatory hyperpigmentation is often transient. These changes are more marked in coloured skins and such patients must always be warned of this potential side effect. Headache of a migraine type is not uncommon when cryosurgery is used on the forehead, temple and scalp and this may last for many hours. Other potential side effects include neuropathy, ulceration, tendon rupture, alopecia and ectropion.

12.11 Contra-indications to cryosurgery

The most important contra-indication to cryosurgery is the absence of an accurate tissue diagnosis before the commencement of treatment. Where the diagnosis of a skin lesion is in any doubt it is advisable to have histological proof of the diagnosis before proceeding with cryosurgery, as this will destroy the tissue and make subsequent histological diagnosis virtually impossible. A range of other contra-indications include the presence of cryoglobulins, agammaglobulinaemia, multiple myeloma, platelet deficiency, blood dyscrasias, Raynaud's disease, cold urticaria, cold intolerance, pyoderma gangrenosum and collagen vascular diseases.

Bibliography

Bohler-Sommeregger K, Schuller-Petrovic, S, Neumann R, Muller E. Cryosurgery of lentigo maligna. *Plast Reconstr Surg* 1992; 90: 436–40.
Colver GB, Dawber RPR. Tattoo removal using a liquid nitrogen cryospray. *Clin Exp Dermatol* 1984; 9: 364–6.

Colver GB, Dawber RPR. Cyrosurgery—the principles and simple practice. *Clin Exp Dermatol* 1989; 14: 1–6.

Dawber R. Cold kills! *Clin Exp Dermatol* 1988; 13: 137–50.

Dawber R, Colver G, Jackson A. *Cutaneous Cryosurgery. Principles and Clinical Practice*. London: Martin Dunitz Ltd., 1992.

Holt PJ. Cryotherapy for skin cancer: results over a 5-year period using liquid nitrogen cryospray cryosurgery. *Br J Dermatol* 1988; 119: 231–40.

Kuflik EG. Cryosurgery updated. *J Am Acad Dermatol* 1994; 31: 925–44.

Shepherd JP, Dawber RPR. Wound healing and scarring after cryosurgery. *Cryobiology* 1984; 21: 157–69.

Tappero JW, Berger TG, Kaplan LD, Volberding PA, Kahn JO. Cryosurgery for Kaposi's sarcoma associated with acquired immune deficiency syndrome (AIDS): a phase two treatment. *J AIDS* 1991; 4: 839–46.

Zacarian SA. *Cryosurgery for Skin Cancer and Cutaneous Disorders*. St Louis: Mosby, 1985: 283–97.

13 Wound care and postoperative management

13.1 Wound healing processes

Wound healing starts with an acute inflammatory response, established within minutes of tissue injury, which continues for a period of some 3 days. Following tissue injury, platelets, red blood cells and neutrophils are attracted to the damaged area; when platelets come into contact with mature collagen, they become activated and are caused to aggregate. Platelet aggregation in turn leads to thromboplastin release, resulting in cleavage of fibrinogen to fibrin, producing a wound clot and establishing haemostasis. Within 6 h, leucocytes and macrophages start to invade the wound and act to remove tissue debris, ingest bacteria and, through their proteolytic action, break down the fibrin clot, making way for the invasion of fibroblasts and endothelial cells. Wounds formed by destructive means, for example by electrosurgery, cryosurgery or laser surgery, heal more slowly than those created by a scalpel or curette. If the surface clot is allowed to dry out it forms a scab which impedes epithelialisation of wound surface. There is evidence that by keeping the surface occluded and moist with, for example, an antibiotic ointment or occlusive dressing, epithelialisation occurs more rapidly. Epithelial cell migration can occur at a rate of between 0.25 and 0.5 mm/day under ideal conditions.

After the inflammatory reaction in the first 48–72 h, the healing phase is dominated by cellular proliferation. Fibroblasts migrate into the wound, moving along the fibrin, collagen and fibronectin matrix and at about day five, start to synthesise collagen, which is essential for the repair process. The proliferative phase of wound healing continues and is maximal around 8 days, continuing for about 40 days.

The maturation of a wound starts to occur around day seven, as collagen bundles become more densely packed and covalent cross-linking of the collagen bundles begins to occur. As the collagen becomes more insoluble, so the tensile strength of the wound starts to increase and the collagen bundles begin to orientate themselves along the lines of tension within the wound. The laying down of collagen and its removal by proteolytic enzymes is a dynamic process which leads to remodelling within the wound, so that collagen is laid down to provide optimal tensile strength. Wound contraction also commences at about 1 week, which aids in reducing the dermal defect and will eventually decrease the size of the wound area by around 40%. Contraction of an open wound proceeds at a fairly constant rate of between 0.6 and 0.75 mm/day, being faster in rectangular or stellate wounds as compared with circular wounds. Epidermal healing can begin as early as 24 h, with both fibrin and fibronectin providing the matrix for epidermal cell migration. A moist tissue environment greatly accelerates epidermal proliferation, both at the sides of the wound and from appendageal structures which may remain in the wound bed.

Angiogenesis occurs at about the same time as fibroblasts appear, and depends on chemotaxis and endothelial cell proliferation, which is stimulated by factors produced by activated macrophages.

Maturation of the wound continues for over 1 year, but the wound area never regains the strength of the normal surrounding tissue. It is interesting to note that after about 2 weeks following primary closure of a wound with sutures, the surgical wound will have achieved only 3–5% of the original skin strength, and at 2 years the tensile strength of the skin may only have increased up to 20% of that of the original skin. Wounds never gain more than 60–80% of their original strength and this may be achieved only after 12–14 years. Given these facts, it is surprising that more wounds do not dehisce following suture removal, and that stretched scars are not more common.

Wound healing can be classified into two main categories: (i) primary intention healing, which occurs when full thickness wounds are approximated at the time of surgery using a wound closure technique (see Chapter 6); and (ii) healing by secondary intention, which occurs by granulation and epithelialisation, when wounds are left open.

Wound healing is generally impaired in patients with diabetes, nutritional deficiencies or poor circulation, or in the setting of previous radiotherapy or corticosteroid therapy.

13.2 Wound healing by primary intention

When wounds are closed using suture techniques, contraction has only a very small role to play in the wound healing process and the period of epithelialisation is usually short, often less than 24 h, especially if the surface of the wound is moist. If such a wound has to be opened during the first week or 10 days following surgery, for example to evacuate a haematoma, then the wound can be directly resutured with no loss in the increasing tensile strength. There is no need to trim the margins of such a wound before resuturing and, indeed, this is to be discouraged as fibroblasts at the margins remain active and quickly bridge the gap following resuturing.

13.3 Wound healing by secondary intention

There has been some reluctance in the past to use this method of healing to close wounds, on the basis that it may lead to complications, such as bleeding, infection and scarring. However, in appropriate circumstances wounds that have been left to heal by secondary intention may have a cosmetic and functional result which is better than that achieved by more formal methods of closure.

Where removal of a non-melanoma skin cancer has not been proven by horizontal frozen section control and the repair has been carried out using a flap or full thickness skin graft, then a subsequent resection of a recurrence may prove difficult. It is advantageous to allow a wound to heal by secondary intention where reconstruction may be difficult or impossible. The management of such a wound area is usually easy; it requires only a daily dressing with an antibiotic ointment under a non-adherent dressing, which can be carried out either by the patient or by a nurse. Secondary intention healing is usually restricted to: (i) smaller wounds; (ii) wounds that cannot be repaired surgically such as those after curettage and cautery; or (iii) where dehiscence of a surgical wound has occurred following infection or necrosis of a flap.

The most important criterion to take into account in considering whether to leave a wound to heal by secondary intention, is perhaps that of the location of the wound. Generally speaking, wounds on concave surfaces heal better than those on convex surfaces, and specifically concave surfaces around the nose, ear, eye and temple heal with excellent results (Fig. 13.1). Wounds on the flat surfaces of the forehead, anti-helix and eyelids usually heal with satisfactory cosmetic results, while those on the convex surface of the nose, lips, cheek, chin and helix of the ear tend to heal with a less cosmetically acceptable scar. Another consideration in secondary intention healing is what effect the process may have on the function of surrounding tissues. For example, healing of a wound on or below the lower eyelid may lead to ectropion; this can be prevented by making a full thickness excision around the lower lid margin, which includes both skin and conjunctiva, so that the hammock-like contraction of both the skin and conjunctiva tends to return the lid margin to a nearly normal contour. Lesions healing on the inner canthus often do well, especially when they are located symmetrically around the inner canthus such that contraction of the wound does not cause ectropion of either of the puncta. Wounds on the upper eyelid margin usually require surgical repair, and are not amenable to healing by secondary intention. Wounds near the edge of the alar ridge may heal with distortion of the alar margin following wound contraction.

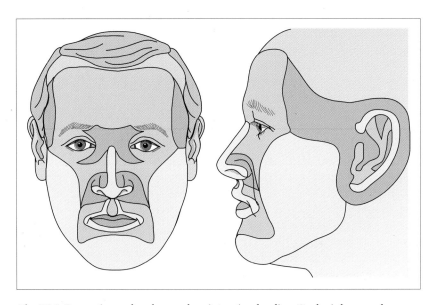

Fig. 13.1 Cosmetic results of secondary intention healing. Dark pink areas show excellent cosmetic results; mid pink areas show satisfactory healing; and pale pink areas show variable cosmetic results.

Wound colonisation with normal skin flora does not seem to interfere with healing, and even light colonisation with pathogenic bacteria seems not to matter much, although frank infection inhibits healing. If a wound shows signs of infection, cleansing twice daily with 3% hydrogen peroxide on sterile gauze before applying a topical antibiotic will usually suffice. It is worth remembering that *Candida albicans* can colonise wounds, especially in a moist environment, and inhibits wound healing. When excess granulation tissue forms, especially in a large wound left to heal by secondary intention, it can usually be dealt with best by gentle curettage, after which wound healing usually proceeds rapidly.

There are a number of other factors that need to be taken into consideration when considering whether or not to allow a wound to heal by secondary intention. Through-and-through defects of the lip, cheek, ala nasi or involving the external auditory canal should be repaired to prevent the formation of fistulae, breathing problems or stenosis. The scar following secondary intention healing is usually hypopigmented, which is acceptable in light coloured skin but may be cosmetically disfiguring in a darkly pigmented patient. Large wounds greater than 6–10 cm in diameter may take months to heal and are liable to break down again after healing has occurred. This seems to particularly apply to wounds on the scalp in the elderly. Wounds with exposed periosteum or perichondrium, or occurring on the lower extremities also heal slowly. By contrast, superficial wounds following curettage and cautery usually heal quite quickly with minimal scarring. In the elderly where skin is lax, contraction caused by secondary intention healing tends to be better camouflaged, and thus the approach is quite appropriate for this group of patients who are often unsuitable candidates for more extensive reconstructive surgery.

Aids to secondary intention healing

On occasion it may be important to direct the line of scar contraction occurring during secondary intention healing; especially around the eye, nose or lip. In these sites 'guiding sutures' can be placed across the wound edges, both to achieve partial skin closure and also to ensure that wound contraction occurs at right angles to the anatomically important border, thus diminishing the risk of possible distortion. Recent work suggests that the use of a collagen sponge, packed into the wound after haemostasis is achieved, may promote secondary intention healing and reduce scar contraction as it provides a matrix for cell migration.

Areas in which bone and cartilage have been exposed by removal of the periosteum and perichondrium will not heal by secondary intention. In the case of cartilage, small perforations can be made, for example on the cartilage of the ear, exposing the perichondrium of the opposite side and allowing granulation tissue to proceed through these perforations (Fig. 13.2). Where the wound overlies bone, it is necessary to remove small areas of the outer cortex of the bone, which will again allow granulation formation and normal wound healing. Alternatively, for wounds of less than about 1 cm in diameter, the outer cortex of the bone may be fenestrated using bone drills, and irrigated with saline to prevent excessive thermal damage. These

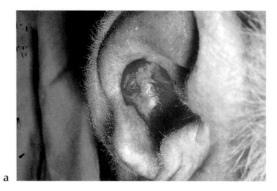

a

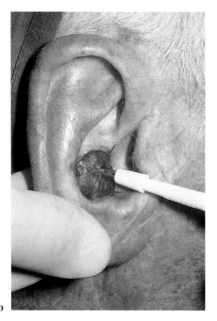

b

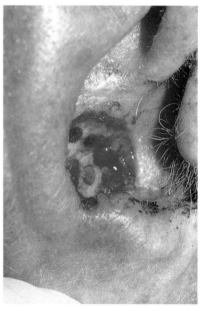

c

Fig. 13.2 Promotion of secondary intention healing over cartilage. **a**. Defect and **b**, **c**. punch excisions of cartilage to stimulate epithelialisation.

processes may not be required as granulation from the edges of the wound would normally be sufficient.

For granulating wounds, an alginate dressing (see below) can be used at the time of surgery to promote coagulation from the capillary bed (Fig. 13.3b). This dressing separates from the wound, with the use of normal saline after 1–3 days, at which stage the wound may be cleaned with 3% hydrogen peroxide, which removes tissue debris and bacteria. The wound can then be dressed and kept moist with an antibiotic ointment (Fig. 13.3d) under a non-adherent bandage (Fig. 13.3e); this treatment is repeated daily until the wound has healed. The appearance of a healing wound improves over 6–12 months with lightening of the colour of the wound as well as softening of its texture; the latter can be promoted by massaging the wound with a massage oil or moisturiser.

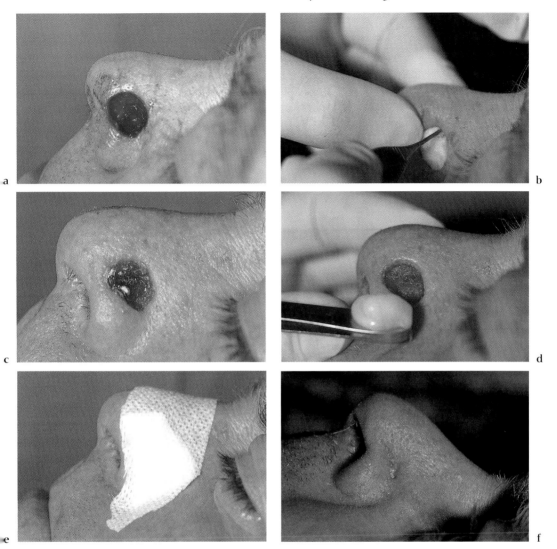

Fig. 13.3 Secondary intention healing. **a**. Defect created at time of surgery.
b. Wound packed with alginate dressing. **c**. Wound at 1 week. **d**. Application of
antibiotic at 1 week. **e**. Non-adherent layer under adhesive dressing. **f**. Wound at 6
weeks.

13.4 Wound dressings for dermatological surgery

Concept of the ideal dressing

The ideal characteristics for a good wound dressing are that: (i) it should aid
in haemostasis; (ii) provide a moist wound surface yet not lead to macera-
tion; (iii) prevent infection and the penetration of foreign material; and (iv)
at the same time absorb away exudate from the wound thus decreasing the

chances of infection. The ideal dressing should also act as a cushion to the wound, preventing trauma, and also limit the amount of movement in the tissue surrounding the wound. Research has shown that the best single form of dressing would be a semi-occlusive one, which allows the wound exudate to pass out while enabling oxygen to penetrate through and aid wound healing.

It is clear that no single dressing meets all the requirements and indeed it is probably not possible to develop such an ideal dressing in view of the different requirements in disparate wounds. The concept has emerged of a layered wound dressing which has a number of layers, each of varying materials, and contributing to the various requirements of a particular wound (Fig. 13.4).

13.5 The layered dressing

The contact layer

Research and the known physiology of wound healing indicate that it is necessary to keep the wound hydrated, to prevent tissue desiccation and encourage epithelialisation of the surface. The stages in dressing a simple wound are illustrated in Figs 13.5–13.8. Perhaps the best way of achieving this goal is to apply an antibiotic ointment to the wound surface as a first layer (see Fig. 13.6).

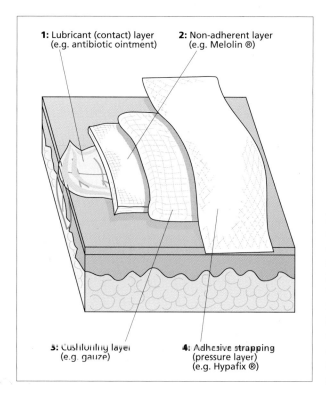

1: Lubricant (contact) layer (e.g. antibiotic ointment)

2: Non-adherent layer (e.g. Melolin ®)

3: Cushioning layer (e.g. gauze)

4: Adhesive strapping (pressure layer) (e.g. Hypafix ®)

Fig. 13.4 The concept of an ideal dressing for a sutured wound. For a non-sutured wound, dressing may be modified by having a contact layer of either antibiotic ointment or alginate dressing.

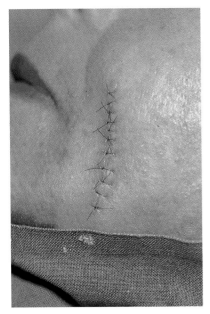

Fig. 13.5 Sutured wound prior to dressing.

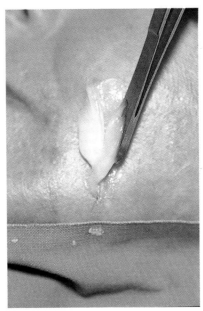

Fig. 13.6 Antibiotic ointment being applied to wound surface.

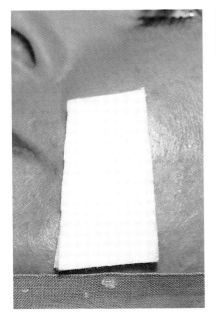

Fig. 13.7 Non-adhesive dressing layer applied to wound.

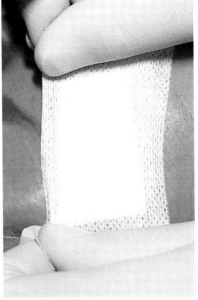

Fig. 13.8 Adhesive layer completes wound dressing.

Such ointments (e.g. Bactroban®, Polyfax® and Fucidin®) act to keep the wound hydrated yet not too occluded, although probably do little to decrease wound infection. An alternative to antibiotic ointments is medicated tulle dressings; here, a gauze dressing has been impregnated with soft white paraffin (Jelonet®, Paratulle®), or with antibiotics such as framycetin (Sofratulle®), or 2% sodium fusidate (Fucidin Intertulle®), or with an antiseptic agent such as chlorhexidine (Bactigras®) or povidone iodine (Inadine®). These greasy, semi-occlusive tulle dressings have a low adherence to the wound, can be used to pack small cavities, and are readily mouldable, allowing them to be adapted to the physical configuration of the wound.

Disadvantages of tulle dressings include some adherence to the wound with possible disruption of the wound on their removal, and the possibility of allergic contact dermatitis to the medicaments in such dressings. Alternative contact dressings are the hydrocolloid dressings (Granuflex®, Comfeel®, Tielle®, Tegasorb®), which prevent entry of infection while promoting a moist environment which encourages granulation and reduces pain, especially in wounds requiring debridement. They are particularly suited to the treatment of leg ulcers, but have also been used in surgical granulating wounds where they have been noted to accelerate healing. The main problem with their use relates to the leakage of malodorous fluid if they are applied to heavily exudating wounds, although this is claimed to be reduced with newer products (Tielle®, Granuflex E®).

Haemostatic agents for secondary intention healing

If there is a tendency for the wound to bleed then it can be dressed with alginate dressings (Kaltostat® (Fig. 13.9), Sorbsan®, Tegagel® or Ultraplast®) as the first layer. Sodium alginate is extracted from seaweed and is soluble in water, while its calcium salt is insoluble. In the manufacture of alginate fibre dressings, calcium and sodium alginate salts are used to form a non-woven fibrous mat. The calcium ions stimulate both platelet aggregation and blood coagulation. These dressings also absorb exudate and tissue fluid and form a hydrophilic gel over the surface of the wound, providing a moist wound environment which promotes wound healing. The dressings largely disintegrate with time, but any remaining portions can be easily removed by irrigation with sterile saline without damage to new wound tissue. Any alginate fibres that get caught

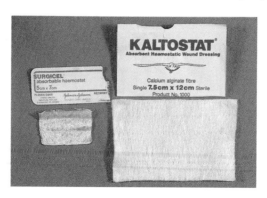

Fig. 13.9 Two commonly used absorbable haemostatic wound dressings. An alginate and oxidised cellulose are illustrated.

up in the granulation tissue are gradually absorbed and do not cause any subsequent problems.

An alternative type of haemostatic dressing is composed of oxidised cellulose; a soft smooth fabric which swells when saturated with blood, producing pressure on the wound which aids haemostasis. It has also been shown to possess anti-bacterial properties. Examples are Surgicel® (Fig. 13.9) and Oxycel®. A variation is the gelatine sponge Gelfoam®, which is a water-insoluble foamed gelatin capable of absorbing many times its weight of blood; it also acts as a haemostat by facilitating thromboplastin release. Gelatin sponges are digested by proteolytic enzymes over a period of 6 weeks, but have the disadvantage that they can promote, rather than inhibit infection. Microfibrillar collagen dressings (Fibracol® (Fig. 13.10)) are relatively new and consist of a water-soluble collagen dressing which may not only act as a haemostat but also as an effective promoter of wound repair.

Non-adherent layer

It is important that the dressing layer in contact with the wound is not only non-adherent, so that when it is removed it does not avulse newly formed epithelium, but that it should also be capable of letting the exudate pass through. Other popular dressings for this layer are the so-called knitted vicrose primary dressings such as N-A® dressing, silicone N-A® dressing and Tricotex®. A number of absorbent dressings have been produced which incorporate a permeable plastic film on one side, to prevent the dressing adhering to the wound, bonded to an absorbent layer, such as Melolin®.

Absorbent layer

An absorbent layer is important in any wound that has an exudate. This layer will generally consist of gauze pads or cotton balls and serves to wick away exudate from the wound surface, thus preventing it from becoming a culture medium for bacteria and deterring crust formations on the wound. If a lot of wound exudate is expected then the composite dressing pad known as 'Gamgee' can be used.

The dressing must be changed once it has become saturated with exudate. The absorbent layer also acts to transmit and distribute pressure from

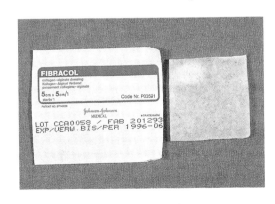

Fig. 13.10 Microfibular collagen wound dressing (Fibracol®) to promote haemostasis and wound healing.

the overlying pressure dressing in a uniform fashion over the wound surface.

Contouring layer

A contouring layer may be necessary in certain instances to fill anatomical depressions such that compression from the next layer can be distributed uniformly over the wound. The contouring layer is most frequently required around the nose and ears. It can be made from such materials as dry gauze pads, fluffed up cotton balls or dental rolls. For example, a gauze dental roll can be used to fill in a nasolabial depression, or gauze can be applied both behind and in front of the ear and held in place with bandaging encircling the head.

Pressure layer

The pressure application layer provides pressure on the wound, collapsing dead space, aiding haemostasis, preventing swelling of the wound and immobilising the area. It also serves to hold the rest of the dressing in place and can be considered as the securing layer. For small wounds not requiring most of the layers, small elastic adhesive bandages may be adequate; these include Elastoplast® and Cutiplast®. If these dressings do not have a non-adherent pad in the centre, one can be fashioned out of a small section of gauze or non-adherent dressing. It is important to ask all patients if they have shown an allergic response to dressings in the past before using these preparations. In the case of Elastoplast® allergy the allergen will usually be colophony; Hypafix® or Mefix® which has an acrylic adhesive system can generally be used in such patients. Conversely, if the patient has a history of sensitivity to acrylic adhesives then Elastoplast® is a better alternative. Hypafix® (Fig. 13.11) and Fixamol® are non-woven polyester fabric-coated dressings which are useful in retaining dressings and providing compression on awkward body contours. The several layers of a dressing on large wounds are best held in place using an adhesive tape, such as conventional non-backed Elastoplast®, or for those who are allergic to this preparation, Scanpore® or Micropore® tape. The disadvantage of these tapes is that they do not stick as well to the skin

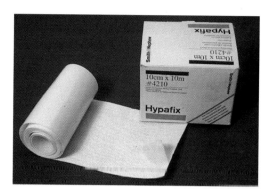

Fig. 13.11 Acrylic adhesive bandage (Hypafix®) for pressure application and securing wound.

initially; they become more adherent several minutes later when they absorb skin surface oils. Further compression to the wound can be applied using, for example, a crepe bandage around the head or cohesive bandages (e.g. Secure Forte®) which adhere to themselves, thus preventing stripping of overlapping turns; they are particularly useful for high-tension dressings on limbs.

It is not always necessary to have all of the layers in the composite bandage as described above. For example, a small excision on the face or limb may simply be covered by an ordinary Elastoplast® bandage, while a more complex flap on the forehead may require all the layers to achieve the maximum benefit from the dressing. A full layer type of dressing can usually be removed at 48 h, after which compression of the wound is not usually required. The wound may then simply be dressed by antibiotic ointment under a non-adherent dressing, or left open until the sutures have been removed.

13.6 Dressings for particular sites

Some areas of the body present particular difficulties with regard to the application of a dressing.

Digits and hands

Because the vascular supply to the digits may be impeded by an enclosing dressing it is best to apply gauze under tape that does not directly encircle the digit. Where it is desirable to apply some pressure to a wound, Melolin® held in place firmly but not tightly by tape can in turn be covered by a tubular bandage of a knitted lightweight fabric (Tubinette®), applied using a fingerstall (Fig. 13.12). It is very important to elevate a limb following surgery to hands, feet and digits to minimise postoperative oedema. It is also important to remember to tell patients who are going to have layered dressings applied to the foot that they will not be able to get their foot into a normal shoe, and that therefore a loose fitting shoe will be required for the journey home!

For hand surgery, elevation can be achieved by using a collar-and-cuff-type sling.

Scalp

Application of dressings to the scalp is difficult because the presence of hair prevents taping of dressings to the scalp; in many cases a dressing may not be required. If pressure is required, then wrapping the whole scalp in a turban-type crepe dressing is necessary. Alternatively, scalp dressings can be held in place using an elastic net or Stockinette® dressing. If pressure is not required on the scalp, then flexible collodion, an antibiotic applied frequently, or semi-permeable film dressings applied as sprays, can be used. Of the latter, two are worth noting: Opsite spray® which consists of methacrylate polymers dissolved in a mixture of ethyl acetate and acetone; and Nobecutane spray® (Fig. 13.13), which is a solution of acrylate resins dis-

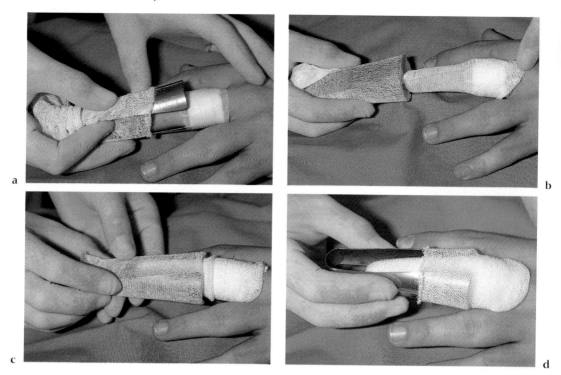

Fig. 13.12 Tubular bandaging being applied to finger using fingerstall.

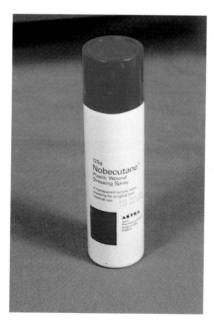

Fig. 13.13 Nobecutane® spray suitable for scalp wounds.

solved in ethyl acetate. After spraying on skin, these dry to form a tough protective film which is impervious to bacteria.

Eye

Following surgical intervention to the eye which has included the use of topical anaesthetic drops, it is advisable that the conjunctiva be covered with an antibiotic ointment (e.g. Chloromycetin®) and the eye closed using an eye pad until sensation returns. The securing tape should be applied from the forehead to the zygoma region.

13.7 Duration of dressing

The time that the initial dressing should be left in place will vary according to the type of wound and the procedure carried out. For example, for a sutured wound the dressing may be changed after 48 h, while for more complicated wounds such as grafts or flaps the surgeon may wish the dressing to remain undisturbed until the next clinic appointment.

For secondary intention healing, the primary dressing may be left on for 48–72 h and then changed on alternate days.

13.8 Wound care when the dressing is removed

When the dressing is removed and it is deemed that the wound is no longer producing an exudate, it may not require further dressing. However, for optimal wound healing the wound should be kept moist with an antibiotic ointment and should be cleaned with sterile saline or 3% hydrogen peroxide to remove scabs and congealed exudate. When the dressing has been removed, the patient may bathe normally, allowing the wound to get wet and simply patting it dry following bathing. At this stage, a thin layer of antibiotic ointment may again be applied.

Bibliography

Eaglstein WH. The genesis of wound repair. In: Thiers B, Dobson R, eds. *The Pathogenesis of Skin Disease*. New York: Churchill Livingstone, 1985: 617–23.

Falanga V, Zitelli JA, Eaglestein WH. Wound healing—periodic synopsis. *J Am Acad Dermatol* 1988; 19: 559–63.

Glasgold MJ, Glasgold A, Silver FH. The use of collagen matrix to enhance closure of facial defects. *Ear Nose Throat J* 1991; 70: 531–7.

Katz S, McGinley R, Leyden JJ. Semipermeable occlusive dressings. *Arch Dermatol* 1986; 122: 58–62.

Latenser J, Snow SN, Mohs FE, Weltman R, Hruza G. Power drills to fenestrate exposed bone to stimulate wound healing. *J Dermatol Surg Oncol* 1991; 17: 265–70.

Nemeth AJ. Wound healing. *Dermatol Clin* 1993; 11: 629–821.

Nemeth AJ, Eaglstein WH, Taylor JR, Peerson LJ, Falanga V. Faster healing and less pain in skin biopsy sites treated with an occlusive dressing. *Arch Dermatol* 1991; 127: 1679–83.

Thomas S. *Wound Management and Dressings*. London: The Pharmaceutical Press, 1990.

Winton GB, Salasche SJ. Wound dressings for dermatologic surgery. *J Am Acad Dermatol* 1985; 13: 1026–44.

Zitelli JA. Wound healing by secondary intention. *J Am Acad Dermatol* 1983; 9: 407–15.

14 Treatment of benign superficial lesions

14.1 Skin tags

Skin tags usually occur as multiple small (1–2 mm) soft papules with a connective tissue stalk. Patients often request their removal for cosmetic reasons, or after they have been irritated by jewellery around the neck, or have become inflamed following twisting on their stalk. Their removal is usually quite straightforward, and may be carried out by picking up the lesion and cutting through the base with curved iris scissors (Fig. 14.1) or, alternatively, by cautery with a flat tip. Local anaesthesia is not usually required if scissors are used. If, however, this cannot be tolerated by the patient, a skin refrigerant or anaesthetic spray such as dichlorotetra-fluoroethane can be used. If the refrigerant is flammable then cautery must not be used to control bleeding. Prior application of EMLA® may facilitate hyfrecation cautery of multiple lesions. Bleeding is usually minimal and can be stopped by pressure, aluminium chloride hexahydrate solution (Fig. 14.1c) or, if necessary, light cautery.

14.2 Seborrhoeic warts

Seborrhoeic warts (basal cell papillomas) occur primarily on the trunk or head and neck of the elderly. They are usually brown or black in colour, sharply demarcated and have the appearance of being 'stuck on' the skin. Seborrhoeic warts can be treated, when they are relatively few in number, by curettage, if necessary under local anaesthesia. Haemostasis can be achieved with aluminium chloride hexahydrate solution or by light cautery or hyfrecation. If the lesion is resistant to removal by simple curettage, the tissue of the seborrhoeic wart can be softened by cautery or hyfrecation. An alternative is to shave seborrhoeic warts off the skin and seal any bleeding vessels using aluminium chloride hexahydrate solution.

When curettage or shave removal of numerous seborrhoeic warts may be impractical, cryotherapy is often extremely useful (Fig. 14.2). Patients will allow 20–30 seborrhoeic warts to be treated on one occasion usually with one freeze–thaw cycle of 15 s each. The cosmetic result of the removal of seborrhoeic warts by any of these methods is good, although hyperpigmentation may occur, especially with large seborrhoeic warts.

14.3 Dermatosis papulosa nigra

Dermatosis papulosa nigra is a common condition occurring in black and Oriental people around the eyes, cheeks and temples. It is characterised by numerous hyperpigmented papules and tags on the face and/or neck. These can usually be easily removed from the skin by snipping off their base

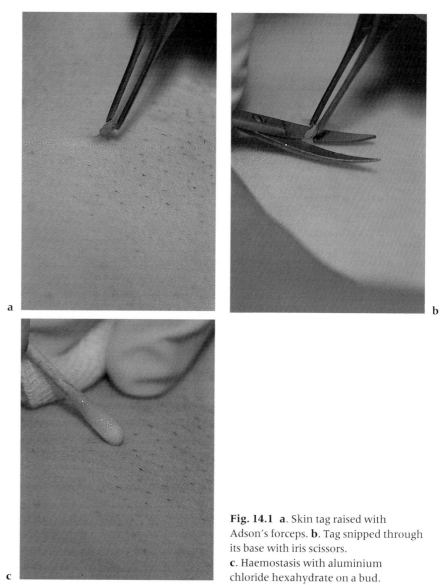

a

b

c

Fig. 14.1 a. Skin tag raised with Adson's forceps. **b**. Tag snipped through its base with iris scissors. **c**. Haemostasis with aluminium chloride hexahydrate on a bud.

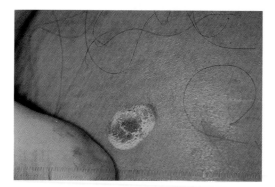

Fig. 14.2 Seborrhoeic wart being treated with liquid nitrogen.

with curved iris scissors, or charring quickly by touching with hot cautery, or a hyfrecator tip or by using light curettage. All of these methods have the major disadvantage of leading to hypo- or hyperpigmentation which can be distressing for patients with pigmented skins; they must be warned in advance.

14.4 Milia

Milia are small inclusion cysts, 1–2 mm in diameter, which appear as white or yellow papules on the face, particularly on the cheeks and eyelids. Milia may be treated by nicking the overlying skin with the tip of a No. 11 blade or a small gauge needle, after which they can usually be extracted by simple pressure, preferably using a comedone extractor.

Alternatively, the skin overlying the milia can be touched by a dull red cautery tip or hyfrecator set at low current. These methods, if used correctly, should not result in scarring.

14.5 Syringoma

Syringomata are yellow to flesh-coloured papules most often occurring in women around the lower eyelids in a symmetrical fashion. Other potential areas of involvement are cheeks, neck, axilla and chest, and an eruptive form can occur on the chest and abdomen. They are hamartomas of the sweat ducts.

If lesions are few in number, excision using curved iris scissors may be possible. Alternatively, they may be desiccated by cautery, or use of the hyfrecator or carbon dioxide laser. Each of these treatments has the disadvantage of leaving small scars.

14.6 Spider naevi

Spider naevi (Fig. 14.3) are probably best treated by gentle use of a hyfrecator set at low power, using the hyfrecator tip to pencil over the central vessel; this technique seldom leads to significant scarring. Cautery may also be used, with the cautery at a low setting, or using a cold point cautery tip. This, however, has the potential disadvantage of leaving a small white scar;

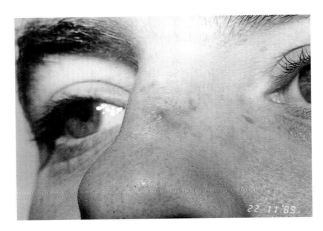

Fig. 14.3 Spider naevus.

the patient must be warned about potential scarring before the procedure is undertaken. For these electrodesiccation methods anaesthesia may obliterate the lesion.

For larger naevi, these methods are not likely to be effective without the risk of significant scarring. In such instances, the use of a pulsed dye laser is likely to give the best results. Occasionally, the central vessel can be removed using a 2-mm punch excision, but this has the obvious disadvantage of replacing the naevus with a scar.

14.7 Campbell De Morgan spots (cherry angiomas)

These 2–5 mm benign red lesions, occurring at mid-life on the upper trunk and arms, are common and represent ectatic blood vessels. They can be treated with cautery or hyfrecation at low power, or can be removed by shave excision, followed by either light cautery or aluminium chloride hexahydrate to achieve haemostasis.

14.8 Facial telangiectasia

Some patients wish to have treatment of small linear facial telangiectases. These often respond well to a tunable dye laser; smaller red vessels respond better than larger blue vessels. Post-inflammatory hyperpigmentation and atrophy are possible side effects. Protection against solar damage to the skin is also to be advised as this can cause or accentuate facial telangiectasia.

14.9 Melanocytic naevi

Melanocytic naevi appear as flat, slightly elevated papillomas or dome-shaped lesions and may be either pigmented or non-pigmented. Clearly, if there is any suggestion that the lesion has undergone recent significant change it should be treated as a melanoma, and this subject is dealt with in Chapter 17.

Removal of a benign cellular naevus for cosmetic reasons or in the case of potential trauma from clothing can usually be undertaken fairly simply. Shave excision (see Chapter 11) is most suitable for naevi that have a dome-shaped elevation (intradermal naevi) and usually produces excellent cosmetic results. The patient should be warned of the possibility of irregular pigmentation in the scar, that future elevation may occur if the naevus is still increasing in size and also that terminal hairs will not be removed. Should these complications occur causing concern, the lesion can subsequently be excised. Another potential difficulty with shave excision of naevi is that the resulting scarring may make histological differentiation from a melanoma more difficult if the lesion has to be excised at a later stage. Alternatively, simple excision of the mole can be carried out provided the naevus has not undergone recent change; the margin beyond the clinical lesion can be kept small. The patient must be clearly warned about the likely size of the scar and about the potential for keloid scarring.

14.10 Xanthelasma

Xanthelasma occur as solitary or multiple yellow cholesterol-containing plaques on or around the eyelids; they only rarely indicate systemic disease

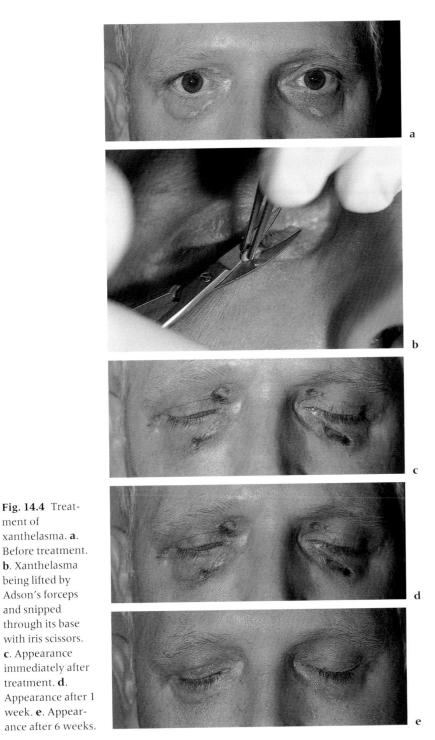

Fig. 14.4 Treatment of xanthelasma. **a**. Before treatment. **b**. Xanthelasma being lifted by Adson's forceps and snipped through its base with iris scissors. **c**. Appearance immediately after treatment. **d**. Appearance after 1 week. **e**. Appearance after 6 weeks.

145

such as hyperlipidaemia. One of the best ways of treating xanthelasma of the upper eyelid is excision under local anaesthesia by lifting them with Adson's forceps and snipping through their base using curved iris scissors. The resultant small wound may then be left to heal by secondary intention with a topical antibiotic being applied by the patient (Fig. 14.4). Care must be exercised on the lower lid so that not too much tissue is removed in order to prevent ectropion.

A time-honoured way of treating xanthelasma is the use of 35–80% trichloroacetic acid to peel the overlying skin. The trichloroacetic acid is carefully applied to the plaque, using an orange stick, until deep frosting occurs. The trichloroacetic acid should then be removed, usually with cotton gauze soaked in water. The area will become ulcerated and form crusts in 10 days to 2 weeks after which healing will occur. The treatment often requires to be applied on several occasions before the xanthelasma is totally cleared. Alternatively, overlying epithelium can be burnt off using light cautery or hyfrecation and the wound left to heal by secondary intention.

14.11 Actinic keratoses

Actinic keratoses are usually multiple, appearing on sun-exposed areas of the skin of elderly people, especially those of fair complexion. They occur most frequently on the face, forehead and scalp and on the dorsa of hands and forearms. Left untreated, the scale can build up to form a cutaneous horn, the base of which may develop into a squamous carcinoma. The histology of an actinic keratosis is that of dysplasia confined to the epidermis. There are several modes of treatment for actinic keratoses and cutaneous horns, depending on the thickness of the lesions, their number and whether or not they have been felt to undergo malignant change. If there are only a few lesions, actinic keratoses are probably best treated with curettage and cautery (Fig. 14.5), which allows the submission of material for histopathology. This is particularly necessary when a cutaneous horn is present, to exclude squamous carcinoma. If carcinomatous change does exist at the base of a cutaneous horn, then definitive excision is required.

If the lesions are more superficial and numerous, then either cryosurgery or topical 5-fluorouracil can be used. Neither of these treatments have the advantage of allowing histological diagnosis, but this is often not required. For cryosurgery (Fig. 14.6) a freeze–thaw cycle of 15–20 s is usually adequate and achieves a cure rate of around 95%.

Topical 5-fluorouracil in the form of a 5% cream (Efudix®) is useful in treating multiple actinic keratosis over larger areas. The 5-fluorouracil causes marked inflammation in both clinically apparent and inapparent lesions. The cream can usually be applied twice daily for up to 3 weeks, during which time the keratosis will become red, inflamed and on occasions, ulcerated. Patients must be warned that if ulceration occurs they should stop the treatment for a few days and apply a topical antiseptic or antibiotic cream. Areas such as the eyelids, vermilion border of the lip and nasolabial areas are particularly sensitive to 5-flourouracil, and are not suitable for this treatment; its inflammatory action is potentiated by sun exposure.

An alternative approach for a patient with multiple solar keratoses, espe-

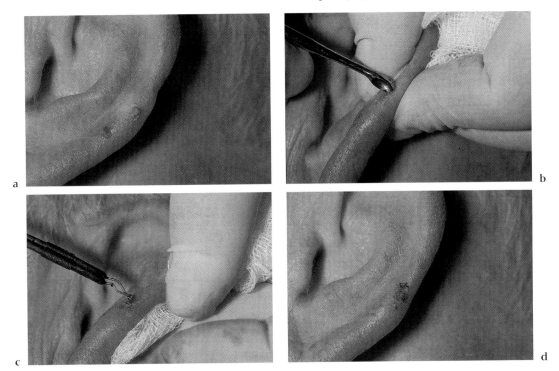

a b c d

Fig. 14.5 Keratosis on ear for curettage and cautery. **a**. Before treatment.
b. Lesion being curetted from skin. **c**. Cautery being applied to base.
d. Wound at end of procedure.

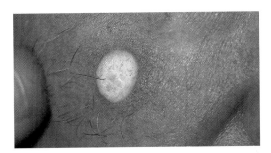

Fig. 14.6 Keratosis treated
with cryosurgery.

cially over the face and scalp areas, is to consider a resurfacing procedure
(chemical peel, laser peel or dermabrasion), both to stop recurrence of new
lesions and to treat those that are already present. This is dealt with in
greater detail in Chapter 19.

14.12 Dermatofibromas

Dermatofibromas are common lesions consisting of firm, smooth, often
hyperpigmented nodules occurring on the limbs, especially in females.
Occasionally, they can be elevated and pruritic, which may cause the
patient to seek medical attention. More often they are asymptomatic, other
than causing concern about the possibility of skin cancer. The patient can
usually be reassured that they are benign in nature and that it is best to

leave them without further intervention. Excision is the only way of removing them, and may result in a worse cosmetic result. Patients wishing to have these lesions removed must therefore be counselled very carefully. Dermatofibromas that are pruritic and pigmented can often be softened, and the symptoms eased, by cryotherapy.

14.13 Sebaceous hyperplasia

Sebaceous hyperplasia consists of creamy pink or yellow-coloured papules, usually occurring on the face, particularly on the forehead and cheeks, in later life or following excessive solar exposure. These lesions can usually best be treated with cryotherapy using a 10–15 s freeze–thaw cycle, preferably using a cotton bud. Other methods include curettage, which will leave a scar, or deep chemical peeling, which may have to be carried out on a number of occasions.

14.14 Verrucous epidermal naevi

Epidermal naevi can be either of the localised or more generalised form, and may have a linear distribution. Histologically they show acanthosis, hyperkeratosis and papillomatosis. Because of the dermal component, it may be difficult to remove epidermal naevi without leaving some degree of scarring. Superficial shaving can be extremely helpful (Fig. 14.7). Electrodesiccation and cryosurgery are also sometimes helpful, as is laser excision which has the advantage of limited injury to the surrounding tissue.

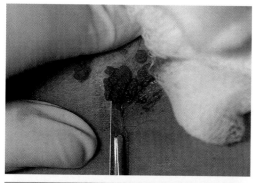
a

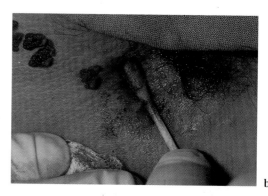
b

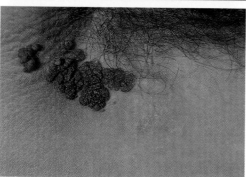
c

Fig. 14.7 a. Treatment of epidermal verrucous naevus by shave biopsy.
b. Aluminium chloride hexahydrate being used for haemostasis. **c.** Healing of area after 3 weeks.

Clearly, if the naevus is small, surgical vaporisation may be definitive, but unfortunately these naevi are usually large and widespread and in such instances excision can lead to a cosmetic result that is worse than the naevus itself.

14.15 Lipomas

A lipoma is a rounded soft tumour which may occur on any part of the body and which can reach sizes of more than 5 cm. Lipomas are the most common of the soft tissue tumours, and although usually located in the subdermal fat, they can occur in deeper structures such as muscle. If lipomas are small and superficial they can occasionally be removed by making a small incision overlying the lipoma, which can then be extruded through the incision by compressing it between the thumb and forefinger, and subsequently cut free. If this method is used the site must be palpated for residual lipoma tissue and haemostasis achieved in the cavity left by the lipoma, as haematoma formation is common.

For a larger lipoma, simple excision is usually better; it must be realised that more tissue than expected may need to be removed as lipomas tend to extend beyond their clinical borders. After the incision is made over the lipoma its nodules can be dissected free using undermining scissors. Again, it is important to achieve good haemostasis, and absorbable sutures may be required to close the considerable dead space and achieve haemostasis.

Lipomas, either solitary or multiple, may also be removed by liposuction (see Chapter 20).

14.16 Pyogenic granuloma

Pyogenic granuloma is a common vascular tumour appearing as a soft nodule 0.5–1 cm in diameter, often occurring on the forearms and hands in response to trauma. Most pyogenic granulomata can be removed by curettage followed by electrodesiccation of the base (see Chapter 10, Fig. 10.2).

Occasionally, bleeding from the central vessel can be brisk and if this is more vigorous cautery or hyfrecation may be required, which can in turn lead to scarring. As an amelanotic melanoma may occasionally resemble pyogenic granuloma and if there is any doubt about the diagnosis, it is essential that tissue be submitted for histopathology. If the diagnosis is not in doubt then cryosurgery is an alternative, but probably less satisfactory treatment (see Chapter 12).

14.17 Lymphangioma circumscriptum

Lymphangioma circumscriptum usually occurs as grouped vesicles filled with yellowish fluid. They most often occur on the trunk and proximal limbs. The dilated lymph vessels in the upper dermis communicate with channels extending to the subcutaneous fat, and even when extensive excision is carried out recurrences are extremely common. The extent of such lesions can now be more accurately assessed using nuclear magnetic imaging techniques. It is usually best not to advise surgery; when it is carried out it needs to be much more extensive than might be anticipated from the clinical appearance of the lesion. There is some evidence that the use of the carbon dioxide laser is helpful in the removal of these lesions, but successful treatment depends upon the vaporisation of the entire lesion.

The pulsed tunable dye laser has been reported recently to be of use in the treatment of angioma circumscriptum, especially when there is some redness due to haemoglobin. Response rates appear to be better than for the carbon dioxide laser.

14.18 Chondrodermatitis nodularis helicis

Chondrodermatitis nodularis helicis (Fig. 14.8) is a common inflammatory condition affecting the cartilage of the external ear, which produces a painful nodule, usually located on the outer rim of the helix. Its precise cause is unknown, but it usually presents with the patient complaining of pain on sleeping on the same side as the lesion, which has led to the theory that it may be caused by tissue ischaemia.

It is estimated that about 25% of early cases will be significantly improved by intralesional corticosteroid. It is probably best to start with intralesional triamcinolone 10 mg/ml injected into the subcutaneous tissues around the inflamed or ulcerated area. This should not be repeated for at least 6 weeks for fear of causing steroid-induced cartilage necrosis. Cryosurgery has also been advocated for this condition but relapse rates can be high.

If surgery is required, two possibilities exist. One is to carry out a wedge resection of the area involved (see Chapter 20) which is usually curative.

An alternative method of treatment has been described, where cartilage alone is resected without the removal of any of the overlying skin, thereby giving a good cosmetic result. In this procedure a flap of skin is raised to

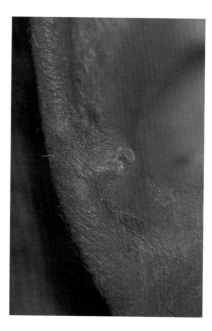

Fig. 14.8 Chondrodermatitis nodularis helicis.

reveal the underlying perichondrium and cartilage of the helix. The cartilage is then carefully trimmed to remove the area of cartilage beneath the ulcer, to a depth of ≈3 mm; any cartilage left is pared such that the cut edge is smooth to the feel. After haemostasis is achieved the skin edges are resutured into place. The advantages of this technique is that it is quick, provides good cosmetic results and is curative, at long-term follow up, of lesions on the helix in over 80% of cases. Recently, a study has shown some value in the injection of collagen solution (Zyplast®) into the space between the cartilage and the overlying skin, which seems to help by producing a cushioning effect, which reduces the pain. Pre-injection of Zyplast® into the volar aspect of the forearm, as described in Chapter 20, is required to exclude patients allergic to this type of product.

14.19 Acne keloidalis nuchae

Acne keloidalis nuchae is a condition characterised by confluent keloidal papules occurring on the occipital area of the posterior scalp and posterior neck, which is most frequent in black skin.

Conventional treatment of acne keloidalis includes antibiotics, topical and intralesional steroids, cryotherapy and retinoids, although all of these treatment modalities are frequently disappointing. Acne keloidalis does well with excisional surgery, with wound closure being by split skin grafting or primary closure, although the latter has the disadvantage of often leading to quite a stretched scar. Better cosmetic results can usually be obtained by excision, either by carbon dioxide laser or cold-steel surgery, of the posterior aspect of the scalp and hairline, followed by allowing the area to heal by secondary intention.

Bibliography

Dolsky RL, Asken S, Nguyen A. Surgical removal of lipomas by lipo-suction surgery. *Am J Cosmet Surg* 1986; 3: 27–34.

Glenn MJ, Bennett RG, Kelly P. Acne keloidalis nuchae: treatment with excision and secondary-intention healing. *J Am Acad Dermatol* 1995; 33: 243–6.

Gonzalez E, Gange RW, Momtaz KT. Treatment of telangiectases and other benign vascular lesions with the 577 nm pulsed dye laser. *J Am Acad Dermatol* 1992; 27: 220–6.

Greenbaum SS. The treatment of chondrodermatitis nodularis chronica with injectable collagen. *Int J Dermatol* 1991; 30: 291–4.

Hudson-Peakock MJ, Cox HN, Lawrence CM. Longterm effectiveness of cartilage removal for the treatment of chondrodermatitis nodularis. *Br J Dermatol* 1995; 133: 46S.

Kantor GR, Ratz JL, Wheeland RG. Treatment of acne keloidalis nuchae with the CO_2 laser. *J Am Acad Dermatol* 1986; 14: 263–7.

Lawrence CM. The treatment of chondrodermatitis nodularis with cartilage removal alone. *Arch Dermatol* 1991; 127: 530–5.

Marks R, Rennie G, Selwood TS. Malignant transformation of solar keratoses to squamous cell carcinoma. *Lancet* 1988; 1: 795–7.

Stegman SJ, Tromovitch TA, Glogau RG. *Cosmetic Dermatological Surgery.* Chicago: Year Book Medical Publishers, 1990.

15 Treatment of warts

15.1 Plane warts

Plane warts occur as flat-topped papules, most often on the face or
dorsum of the hands of young children and women, and tend to be of
uniform size (3–4 mm in diameter). Almost invariably they occur in multiple clusters and are particularly prone to Köbnerisation along scratch
lines. They often have a slight tan colour or blend in with the colour of
the surrounding skin and can be best seen by tangential lighting. Plane
warts are caused by HPV10 virus and can often persist for many years
before there is spontaneous resolution. Resolution is often preceded by a
sudden increase in the number and size of the lesions. Plane warts are
regarded by many as a minor cosmetic problem; and are probably best left
alone as treatments are largely unsatisfactory. Certainly, aggressive therapy
which may lead to scarring is not warranted for the treatment of plane
warts.

If, however, the patient does wish to have treatment, several modalities
of treatment have been used with varying success.

Perhaps the least aggressive approach is the use of topical tretinoin
(Retin-A® cream) 0.025%, or 1% salicylic acid; both produce a mild peel
and can be applied daily. Alternatively, liquid nitrogen can be applied using
a 5–7 s freeze–thaw cycle; treatments are carried out at weekly or fort-
nightly intervals. Care needs to be taken, especially when treating patients
with pigmented skins, to prevent pigmentary changes. Another alternative
is the use of a hyfrecator, set at the minimal output, used with a pointed tip
held 1 mm above the skin. With experience, the operator can remove plain
viral warts with little or no risk of scarring. However, it is probably wise to
start this form of treatment in a small inconspicuous patch before proceeding to cosmetically important areas. Other treatments for plane warts
include use of 5% fluorouracil cream daily, and 10–35% trichloroacetic
acid carefully applied to the lesion and repeated every few weeks; the latter
has the disadvantage of occasionally leading to hypopigmentation.

15.2 Verruca vulgaris

Common warts account for 10–25% of referrals to a dermatologist, and one
recent survey of British schoolchildren suggests that their prevalence is
about 4–5% in teenagers.

Common warts can be subdivided into a number of clinical groups.
Common viral warts are skin coloured or brownish rough elevations which
occur most commonly on the finger (Fig. 15.1), elbows or knees of children
and young adults. When the hyperkeratotic cap is pared away, the whitish
like substance of the wart is revealed with typical black dots of capillary
bleeding, which originates from capillary loops within the wart tissue. A

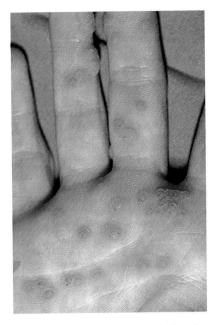
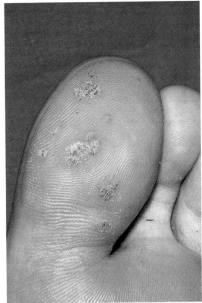

Fig. 15.1 Common warts on the hand. **Fig. 15.2** Mosaic warts on the toe.

variant is the filiform wart, which forms as an elongated outgrowth, frequently solitary, usually on the face and most commonly on the nose of children. Both common and filiform warts rarely give rise to discomfort but have been regarded with distaste since ancient times; their treatment is usually for cosmetic reasons.

By contrast, plantar warts (verrucas) which occur as firm thickenings on the sole, the border of which is often surrounded by a callus like epidermal hypertrophy, are commonly painful and tender especially when they occur on the heel or under the metatarsal heads. A variant of the plantar wart is the mosaic wart, which forms plaque-like lesions which are often extensive and typically occur on the back of the heel, or occasionally on the palms of the hands and around the nails. Mosaic warts (Fig. 15.2) are usually painless but when they become thick they can develop painful fissures. Mosaic warts are typically resistant to most forms of therapy. When treating recalcitrant periungual warts of the hands or feet, or plantar warts, it is worth considering the possibility of such lesions, especially if solitary, being squamous cell carcinomas.

Prognosis

It must be realised that if warts are left alone they will undergo spontaneous regression, with the development of cell-mediated immunity, in anything between 3 months and 5 years, with 20% clearing in 3 months, 50% clearing in 2 years and 93% clearing after 5 years. Warts may undergo regression in a number of different clinical ways including silent shrinkage, swelling and inflammation or haemorrhagic necrosis. It is not uncommon for an increase in the number and size of warts in the weeks prior to their spontaneous remission. Spontaneous remission can be hampered by defects in the immune system as occurs in patients with atopy, patients on immunosuppressive drugs and those with HIV infection.

Topical treatments

The mainstay of therapy for most viral warts in the community is the self application of salicylic acid wart paints, plasters, gels and ointments, a large variety of which are presently on the market. These preparations contain salicylic acid at varying concentration from 10 to 26% and are most frequently dispensed in a collodion-based paint, sometimes combined with lactic acid (Cuplex®, Duofilm®, Salactol®, Salatac®), and which are designed to be applied to the wart tissue each night. More recently, there have been a number of preparations which are dispensed in the form of quick solidifying gel (Salatac®, Occlusal®) and can be more accurately applied, thus preventing spread beyond the wart tissue. The paints can best be applied using a pointed applicator, sharpened matchstick or small brush; if these applicators are used it is sometimes necessary to protect the surrounding skin using Vaseline®. Other topical treatments include formaldehyde (Veracur®) and glutaraldehyde (Glutarol®, Novaruva®, Verucasep®) preparations. Trichloracetic acid 35–80% may be useful for resistant peri-ungual warts.

Of the utmost importance in the treatment of viral warts with topical agents is the removal of excess keratin and dead tissue using a rough pumice stone, emery board or callus file; without this the active ingredient will not reach the wart base, which is necessary if it is to be effective. Soaking the skin until it is soft just prior to the application of the wart paint will also aid absorption. This form of treatment is to be particularly recommended in children as it avoids pain and discomfort associated with cryosurgery.

Used in this way, topical preparations will cure 70–80% of common warts and 80–90% of plantar warts within 3 months. Topical preparations can safely be used on peri-ungual warts and, indeed, for these is probably the treatment of choice. It must be remembered that the topical wart preparations should not be applied to facial skin because of the risk of scarring.

Cryosurgery for verruca vulgaris

Cryosurgery is a simple, quick and efficient method of treating most warts (see Chapter 12) and is increasing in popularity, although it has been shown that the cure rates differ little from those achieved using topical treatments.

Cryosurgery is of use in the treatment of virtually all forms of common warts, but should be used with care on those around the proximal nail fold as damage to the underlying nail matrix may result in permanent nail dystrophy. Treatment of peri-ungual warts, even at the lateral nail fold margin, is often painful because of the oedema induced in the nail bed area. Care must also be exercised in treatment over tendons and nerves where cryotherapy may result in injury to these structures. It should be borne in mind that warts will eventually clear on their own leaving no scarring; treatment should be avoided if it is likely to produce dermal injury and scarring. Scarring is not usually a problem with cryosurgery when the freeze–thaw cycle is less than 30 s.

Cryosurgery to warts can be delivered with either the cotton bud applicator, the Histofreezer® or the spray technique using a cryogun. Before treatment, the wart should be pared as keratin is a good insulator against cold damage. Freezing should continue until frosting extends to 1–2 mm beyond the margin of the wart. The length of the freeze–thaw cycle will depend on the site, thickness and response to previous treatment of the wart but will usually be in the range of 10–30 s. As the effects of liquid nitrogen vary a great deal between patients, it is best to start off with relatively short freeze–thaw cycles, if necessary increasing the duration of the freeze according to the response. The freeze–thaw cycle may be as short as 5 s for plane warts, 10–15 s for hand warts and as much as 30 s for some plantar warts. Filiform warts seem to do particularly well; treatment for as short a time as to bring the wart to a uniform freeze may be effective (Fig. 15.3).

The patient must be warned before treatment of the post-cryotherapy pain and of the possibility of blister formation, and should be instructed to puncture the blister if necessary with a sterile needle, apply an antiseptic or antibiotic ointment and keep the area clean and dry. Treatment with liquid nitrogen can be painful, especially for young children and, except for filiform warts, usually requires more than one treatment. The use of EMLA®

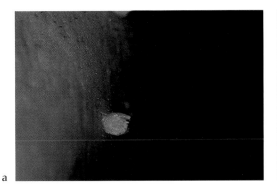

a

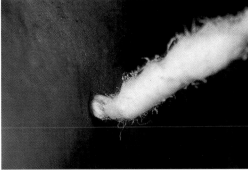

b

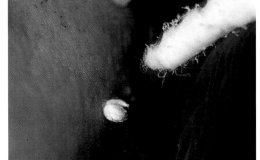

c

Fig. 15.3 Filiform wart being treated with liquid nitrogen by bud technique.

(see Chapter 5), applied 2 h before treatment may reduce pain during the treatment for children, and all patients should be instructed to take paracetamol or aspirin as necessary after cryotherapy. Cryotherapy can be combined with use of topical preparations as soon as inflammation has settled. The interval between treatments should not be greater than 3 weeks as treatment intervals longer than this can reduce the cure rate quite dramatically. The frequency of cryosurgery may range from 1 to 3 weeks, with the cure rate being related more to the total number of treatments given rather than to frequency of treatment. A more rapid cure may therefore be achieved by more frequent treatments. The cryospray has the advantage of making the treatment of multiple warts quicker and more effective, but its use can be frightening for young children, for whom the bud method is usually better tolerated.

Curettage and cautery

Curettage and cautery can be an excellent method of treating warts, especially when they are few in number. After anaesthesia of the area, wart tissue can be softened by application of either cautery or the hyfrecator, making curettage much easier. This is usually not required for filiform-type warts which shell out of the skin fairly easily. Curettage may also be used to advantage when treating peri-ungual warts, which can be removed from under the lateral or distal nail folds, if necessary by paring back the nail plate. A disadvantage of curettage and cautery or the use of a hyfrecator is that vigorous use can lead to scarring.

The treatment of plantar warts requires that the wart surface is pared to reveal the active wart tissue. A No. 15 scalpel blade may then be used to make a vertical incision around the lesion just beyond the junction between the wart and apparently normal tissue. This allows the insertion of a small curette, which is used to remove the wart tissue. Bleeding can be quite vigorous and requires the application of cautery, while keeping the base relatively free of blood through the use of pressure on the surrounding skin. The cavity may then be plugged with a haemostat such as Kaltostat®, before application of a firm dressing (e.g. Melolin® under Hypafix®). After 48 h the patient may dress the wound with an antibiotic ointment under a simple dressing until healed. This technique can, on occasion, lead to a painful scar, and recurrence is a possibility. Mosaic-type plantar warts do not shell out of skin as easily as solitary warts, and cryotherapy may be better for these; it has to be said that no form of therapy is particularly effective for this form of wart.

Light cautery or high-frequency sparking from a hyfrecator can be a useful means of controlling small warts on the beard area.

Patients should be watched for signs of early recurrence as failure to recognise this is one of the most frequent causes for treatment failure.

Excision

Excision of warts using standard surgical techniques is generally not advised because there is a high rate of recurrence in the scar. Filiform warts can be removed by snipping the base with curved iris scissors, and applications of either cautery or aluminium chloride hexahydrate used for haemostasis.

Anogenital warts

The treatment of anogenital warts is best performed in a genito-urinary clinic where other sexually transmitted diseases can be excluded. Anogenital warts may be treated either with topical 20% podophyllin in tincture of benzoin applied weekly or as tolerated at the clinic, or by cryotherapy. Alternatively, podophyllotoxin, the purified active ingredient of podophyllin, and which is significantly less toxic than podophyllin, may be used as a home-based treatment; podophyllotoxin preparations that can be applied by the patient are available (Condyline®, Warticon®). Podophyllin is absorbed from mucosal surfaces and can lead to toxic reactions, local pain and erosions and must be avoided in pregnancy. Anogenital warts in children raise the possibility of sexual abuse which must be excluded by detailed history and examination; this is probably best carried out by a paediatrician with experience in the field.

15.3 Treatment of warts resistant to other modalities of treatment

Lasers

Carbon dioxide lasers are being increasingly used in the treatment of resistant warts (Fig. 15.4). The carbon dioxide laser allows the precise and effective vaporisation of wart tissue and, in experienced hands, damage to the surrounding normal tissue can be minimal. Wart tissue can be vaporised using the defocused beam at low to medium power; small satellite warts

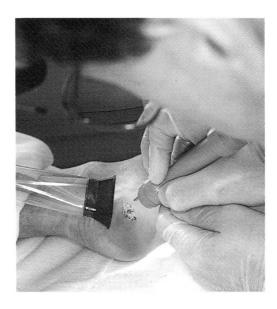

Fig. 15.4 Plantar wart undergoing treatment with the carbon dioxide laser.

can be detected using a binocular loop and treated. The carbon dioxide laser seems to be especially good at treating peri-ungual warts, since it can also be used to vaporise the overlying nail plate if this is required to expose the wart. Warts on mucous membranes and in the anal and genital areas can also be treated in this way. Postoperatively the wound is allowed to heal by granulation. The disadvantages of the carbon dioxide laser are the expense of the laser, the relatively high rate of scarring, postoperative pain and a potential risk to the operator from papilloma virus present in the smoke plume.

Intralesional bleomycin

Bleomycin is a glycopeptide which binds to cellular deoxyribonucleic acid (DNA), resulting in a cytotoxic effect. Intralesional bleomycin may be used in the treatment of warts recalcitrant to other forms of therapy, and is relatively free of complications. Bleomycin is prepared as a 0.1% solution by adding 15 ml of normal saline to 15 mg of bleomycin in a vial, which may then be refrigerated at 4°C for up to 30 days. After cleansing the skin overlying the wart, bleomycin is injected into the wart tissue using a tuberculin syringe fitted with a 35-gauge needle, until there is visible blanching of the wart tissue. As injection can cause moderate pain of short duration, the wart may be anaesthetised first by injection with lignocaine. Multiple injections can be made into larger warts but no more than 0.1 ml should be injected into any one focus within a wart. During the first week following injection, blackening and desiccation of the wart will often become evident. Warts that have not responded to treatment can be reinjected at 4-weekly intervals; the risk of systemic toxicity is deemed to be negligible, provided a maximum total dose of 10 mg is not exceeded. In most cases, healing occurs without scarring. However, episodes of nail dystrophy and persistent Raynaud's phenomenon have occurred following the use of bleomycin for warts on fingers. Its use is contra-indicated in pregnancy and in persons with peripheral vascular disease.

Recently, the use of bleomycin 'pricked' into warts has been described. After anaesthetising the wart with EMLA®, bleomycin solution at a concentration of 1 mg/ml is dropped onto the wart and 'pricked' into it using a Monolet® needle, using approximately 40 punctures per 5 mm^2 of wart tissue. This treatment achieved a 90% clearance of warts after four monthly treatments. This may be a satisfactory way of delivering bleomycin to recalcitrant peri-ungual, mosaic and plantar warts.

Immunotherapy

Most advances in immunotherapy have been disappointing and have not lived up to early expectations. Levamisole and inosine pranobex have been shown to be effective in stimulating the immune system but seem of little use in the treatment of warts. Recently, treatment with cimetidine in doses of 25–40 mg/kg per day for 12 weeks appeared to increase the rate of spontaneous clearance of resistant warts.

The use of dinitrocholorobenzene (DNCB) as a topical sensitiser has been shown to be of value in stimulating the immune system and encouraging spontaneous regression of warts, especially on the palms and soles, but as it has now been shown to be a mutagen, it should not be used. The chemically related compound diphencyprone, which does not appear to be a mutagen, has also been used in the immunotherapy of warts, but as this can lead to recurring eczema, its use cannot be routinely recommended.

Retinoids such as isotretinoin or acitretin have been used as a treatment for extensive recalcitrant viral warts in immunosuppressed patients with varying degrees of success and may be worth considering in immunocompromised patients. However, the retinoids seem only to reduce the hyperkeratosis, and the warts return when the drug is stopped.

Treatments such as interferon-α, interleukin-2 and photodynamic inactivation of wart viruses are still largely experimental.

15.4 Molluscum contagiosum

Molluscum contagiosum is a common condition caused by infection with a pox virus and occurs frequently in young children. Clinically, the lesions appear as small shiny round papules with a small central depression (Fig. 15.5). Most lesions are only a few millimetres in diameter, although more rarely large giant molluscum lesions can achieve sizes of up to 1 cm over 2–3 months. Although lesions of the smaller variety can be profuse, especially in the young and immunosuppressed, in nearly all cases they resolve spontaneously, usually within 1 year. Because of this natural tendency to regression, the possibility of scarring following surgical intervention, and the fear induced in small children by having treatments carried out in hospital, it is often wise to try and convince parents that it is better to leave molluscum alone.

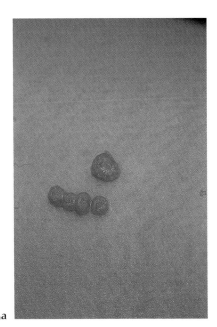 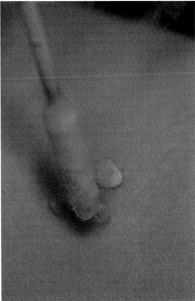

a   b

Fig. 15.5 a. Molluscum contagiosum lesions and **b**. undergoing cryotherapy.

For the treatment of molluscum contagiosum in adults, puncturing of the lesions with a finely pointed toothpick dipped in liquid phenol is often effective in inducing minor inflammation and spontaneous regression. This is not to be recommended in children, who may move during the treatment leading to the dissemination of phenol and subsequent chemical burns. An alternative and easier approach is the use of liquid nitrogen, either applied with a cotton bud (Fig. 15.5) or spray. Usually, only a few seconds of treatment is required to inflame the lesion and induce spontaneous remission. However, even this is not often tolerated by small children, even when using EMLA® for anaesthesia.

A very good alternative for children is the use of topical cantharadin (Cantharone®, currently only readily available in the USA, Fig. 15.6) in a collodion base, which may simply be dabbed onto the lesions using an orange stick. Lesions thus treated should be allowed to dry and must not be covered with a dressing as this may favour blistering. Parents should be warned about the likelihood of blistering. The mollusca become reddened and inflamed over the subsequent few days, but children usually complain of little more than itch. It is probably prudent not to use this treatment on the face or flexural areas.

In children it may be possible to treat a molluscum by puncturing the lesion with a pointed toothpick or orange stick without the use of any caustic material. For those with only a few lesions of molluscum the use of a sharp spoon curette to scoop the lesions from the skin surface may be adequate. Local anaesthesia is not usually required but in children the use of EMLA® as a topical local anaesthetic can be of benefit.

The profusion of molluscum contagiosum occurring in patients taking immunosuppressive drugs or those with AIDS can be difficult to control, and treatment by topical therapies alone may not be effective. In cases of extreme immunosuppression, systemic retinoids have been reported as being of some use.

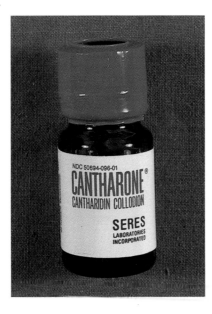

Fig. 15.6 Cantharadin for treatment of molluscum contagiosum.

Bibliography

Bourke JF, Berth-Jones J, Hutchinson PE. Cryotherapy of common viral warts at intervals of 1, 2 and 3 weeks. *Br J Dermatol* 1995; 132: 433–6.

Bunney M, Benton C, Cubie HA. *Viral Warts: Their Biology and Treatment*, 2nd edn. Oxford: Oxford University Press, 1992.

Epstein E. Cantharidin treatment of molluscum contagiosum. *Acta Derm Venereol (Stockh)* 1989; 69: 91–2.

James MP, Collier PM, Aherne W, Hardcastle A, Lovegrove S. Histologic, pharmacologic, and immunocytochemical effects of injection of bleomycin into viral warts. *J Am Acad Dermatol* 1993; 28: 933–7.

Logan RA, Zachary CB. Outcome of carbon dioxide laser therapy for persistent cutaneous viral warts. *Br J Dermatol* 1989; 121: 99–105.

Munn SE, Marshall M, Clement M. A new method of intralesional bleomycin therapy in the treatment of recalcitrant warts. *Br J Dermatol* 1995; 133: 41S.

Orlow SJ, Paller A. Cimetidine therapy for multiple viral warts in children. *J Am Acad Dermatol* 1993; 28: 794–6.

Shelley WB, Shelley ED. Intralesional bleomycin sulfate therapy for warts. A novel bifurcated needle puncture technique. *Arch Dermatol* 1991; 127: 234–6.

Shumack PH, Haddock MJ. Bleomycin: an effective treatment for warts. *Aust J Dermatol* 1979; 20: 41–2.

Street ML, Roenigk RK. Recalcitrant periungual verrucae: the role of carbon dioxide laser vaporization. *J Am Acad Dermatol* 1990; 23: 115–20.

Williams HC, Potter A, Strachan D. The descriptive epidemiology of warts in British shoolchildren. *Br J Dermatol* 1993; 128: 504–11.

16 Cyst removal

One of the most common surgical operations carried out on the skin is that of removal of skin cysts. So-called 'sebaceous cysts' (80% of cysts) on the head, neck and trunk are histologically epidermoid cysts and are associated with a central punctum; pilar cysts (trichilemmal cysts) comprise some 20% of cysts, occur mainly on the scalp and do not have a central punctum. Both forms of cyst present as a smooth fluctuant lump which is often ballottable. In the case of the epidermoid cyst, cheesy foul-smelling material may be expressed from a small punctum.

Patients often request removal of their cystic lesions simply for cosmetic reasons. Another reason for cyst removal is that they are prone to undergo recurrent inflammation or become infected.

16.1 Preoperative assessment

Patients may present with cysts that are red and tender. This can be due either to inflammation following spillage of keratinous cyst contents into the surrounding dermis, or from infection occurring within a long-standing cyst. Infected cysts are usually more painful and erythematous than uninfected inflamed cysts. This distinction is important as inflamed cysts will often resolve with intralesional steroids whereas infected cysts require drainage and systemic antibiotics. It is wise to wait at least 4–6 weeks after the appropriate treatment, until the cyst has become non-tender, before attempting surgical removal.

16.2 Freely movable versus fixed cysts

It is important to assess before operation whether a cyst is freely mobile beneath the skin surface, or whether episodes of inflammation or infection have led to fibrosis, making dissection of the cyst from the surrounding fibrous tissue very difficult. The degree of adherence of the cyst to the surrounding connective tissue can usually be assessed by cyst ballottement (Fig. 16.1). Cysts that have not been previously inflamed will usually move freely under the dermis, whereas cysts in which previous infection has resulted in thick scar formation will usually prove relatively immobile.

Whether or not a cyst is freely mobile dictates the surgical approach; freely movable cysts can usually be shelled out of the skin relatively easily through a small incision, whereas it is probably best to excise the whole fibrous mass around an immobile cyst.

16.3 Operative technique

Scalp cysts

Control of hair is important for ease of removal of scalp cysts. With careful planning it is possible to avoid removing much of the patient's hair, but it is useful to trim a narrow area around the lesion. Removal is best done by clipping, as shaving induces microtrauma to the skin, increasing the chances of postoperative infection. The hair can be held down on either side by adhesive tape or, more conveniently, with a sterile gel, such as KY® jelly which is supplied in small foil sachets suitable for this purpose. An alternative is to use a net-type dressing (Netelast®), with a small opening at the site of surgery to keep hair in place. Alternatively, the hair can be wetted with Hibiclens® scrubbing solution and smoothed down, or held down with an expansile mesh gauze dressing, with a hole cut in it of appropriate size to the surgical field.

Anaesthesia

Before removal of the cyst the overlying and surrounding skin must be anaesthetised. The use of adrenaline in the anaesthetic will greatly decrease the amount of bleeding encountered during the operation, especially on the scalp. Furthermore, the local anaesthetic can often be used to 'hydro-dissect' the cyst from the surrounding connective tissue. The technique involves placing the needle between the overlying skin and the underlying cyst and injecting the anaesthetic into the plane separating the cyst from the surrounding connective tissue, thus delineating this plane for dissection at a later stage (Fig. 16.2).

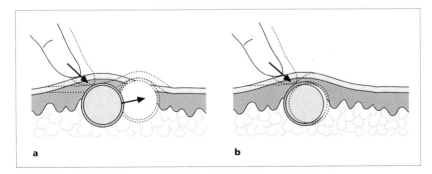

a   b

Fig. 16.1 Assessment of cyst mobility by ballottement.

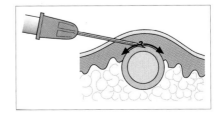

Fig. 16.2 'Hydro-dissection' of cyst using local anaesthetic.

Mobile cysts

Removal of a mobile cyst is best carried out by excising an ellipse of normal skin surrounding the punctum. The skin should be marked using a skin pencil in the form of an ellipse, the long axis of which should lie along the skin tension lines, and should be centred on the punctum of the cyst, if present. The ellipse is then mobilised by incising down to and including the dermis, taking care not to incise the cyst itself if at all possible. The surrounding skin is then raised on a skin hook or with forceps, and the connective tissue around the cyst is gently dissected with either artery forceps or tissue dissecting scissors (Fig. 16.3). When the right plane of dissection has been achieved, the glistening white surface of the cyst will be seen. Dissection is continued down and under the cyst on both sides, until it can be lifted out of the wound by means of grasping its small ellipse of overlying skin. Excision of the overlying small ellipse of skin has the advantage of

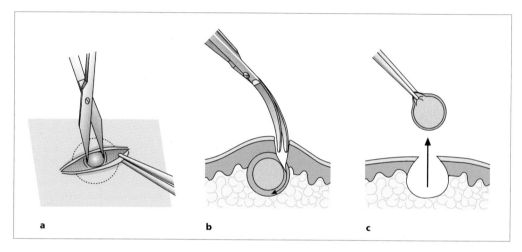

Fig. 16.3 Dissection and removal of mobile cyst.

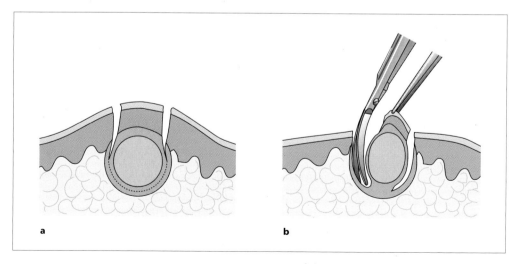

Fig. 16.4 *En bloc* removal of a fixed immobile cyst.

removing excess skin which has developed over the cyst in response to its slow expansion. The amount of excess skin can be judged prior to operation and the size of the ellipse can be planned accordingly. An alternative approach, involving incision of the cyst with manual expression of the cyst contents prior to excision of the residual cyst wall, is advocated by some skin surgeons, but it is not recommended by the authors.

After removal of larger cysts, the dead space in the wound can be considerable. It is important to ensure good haemostasis; deep subcutaneous sutures should be placed, if necessary in layers, to obliterate the dead space. Finally, the skin is closed using subcutaneous sutures to the dermis and interrupted sutures to the skin surface.

Immobile cysts

In the case of cysts that are firmly bound to the surrounding connective tissue, it is usually difficult and sometimes impossible to dissect them free from fibrotic tissue. In such cases it is wiser to mark up a skin ellipse, the central part of which allows deep excision of all fibrotic tissue which includes the cyst (Fig. 16.4). This will usually entail creating an ellipse which is larger than that for mobile cysts, and the wound is often deeper because of the removal of the fibrotic tissue. The wound, however, can be closed using the standard method of buried cutaneous sutures to close dead space, followed by dermal sutures and cutaneous sutures, as described above for mobile cysts.

It is important to send all cysts removed for histopathology, even if the diagnosis seems fairly clear, as there is a very small incidence of basal cell and squamous cell carcinomas arising from epidermoid cysts.

16.4 Wound dressing

In non-hairy areas a pressure dressing should be applied to the area for 48 h, usually in the form of gauze followed by adhesive tape; the resultant pressure decreases the possibility of haematoma formation occurring in any remaining dead space. For cysts on the scalp, dressings involving taping are impractical, and on such areas a semi-permeable, solvent-based film dressing can be useful and may be left in position until the sutures are removed. Solvent-based dressings based on modern synthetic polymers form a tough protective film barrier, discouraging the invasion of the wound by bacteria, while being permeable to water vapour and oxygen but impermeable to water. Examples include Opsite® (ethoxyethyl methacrylate and methoxyethyl methacrylate in ethyl acetate and acetone) and Nobecutane® (acrylic resins in ethyl acetone). A pressure dressing is not usually required on the scalp but, if judged desirable, gauze may be held in place by means of an elastic net or stocking net dressing.

17 Pigmented lesions including melanoma

17.1 Is the lesion a melanoma?

The clinical diagnosis of melanoma may not be easy and an early clinical diagnosis may not be reliable. Many dark lesions are not melanomas and not all melanomas are pigmented (Figs 17.1–17.4, Table 17.1). The clinician is often faced with a pigmented lesion on the skin which he or she considers to be possibly a melanoma but where the diagnosis is by no means certain.

Until recently, the clinical diagnosis of melanoma was based on history and macroscopic visual examination of the lesion. The dermatoscope is increasingly being used in an attempt to improve the accuracy of melanoma diagnosis. The dermatoscope is a hand-held instrument (Fig. 17.5) with a glass footplate and halogen light, which gives a skin surface magnification of about 10. Some experience is necessary for the accurate use of this instrument, but expanded use in dermatology may result in fewer excisions of benign lesions in the future.

17.2 Primary surgical excision

When a lesion is suspected as being a melanoma (Table 17.2), surgical intervention should be undertaken promptly. It is prudent to measure tumour size, record the site, presence or absence of satellite lesions and assess the presence of local lymphadenopathy. Particularly in the case of lentigo maligna, the use of a Wood's light may be helpful in delineating the lesion, which may extend well beyond the margins evident on superficial clinical inspection. A theoretical consideration while performing primary excision of a possible melanoma is that injection of local anaesthetic close to the tumour might cause malignant cells to be dislodged and forced into vascular channels. Although this complication has never been documented, it seems prudent to advise the placement of local anaesthetic some distance from the primary lesion, or to use some form of local nerve block if possible.

There are no data to suggest that incisional biopsy increases the risk of early dissemination, although such biopsies do make full histological assessment difficult, in particular of tumour thickness, on which management depends. The technique of total excision of the lesion with a narrow margin (2 mm) is the best approach when the diagnosis is not certain. This enables the pathologist to make a full assessment of the diagnosis and of the depth of tumour invasion in the case of melanoma, and prevents an unnecessary larger excision if the lesion does not turn out to be a melanoma. Planned definitive surgery in the case of melanoma may then be performed within 2 weeks, and decisions on the width of clearance required can be made in the light of the histological findings on tumour

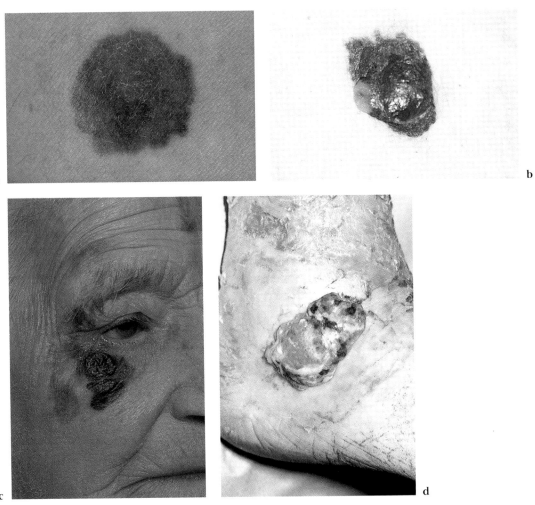

Fig. 17.1 Atlas of melanoma. **a**. Superficial spreading melanoma; **b**. nodular melanoma; **c**. lentigo maligna melanoma; and **d**. amelanotic melanoma.

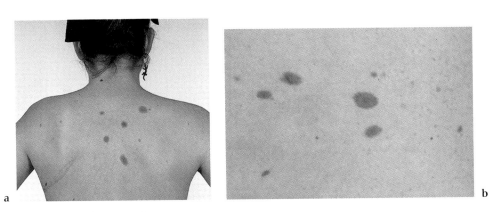

Fig. 17.2 Dysplastic naevi.

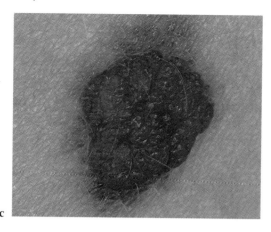

Chapter 17

c   **Fig. 17.2** *Continued*

Table 17.1 The differential diagnosis of melanoma.

Diagnosis	Clinical features
Benign melanocytic naevus	Change in a naevus raises the question of removal for diagnostic purposes
Blue naevus	Dark blue lesion often present from early age and remaining stable throughout life; any change remove
Dysplastic naevus	Atypical pigmented naevus with mottling and irregular margin; often multiple
Ephelis (freckle)	Usually multiple on sun exposed sites; 2–3 mm diameter, tan coloured; darkens on sun exposure
Benign lentigo	5–10 mm diameter; tan to brown in colour; may occur on any skin surface; darkens little on sun exposure
Labial melanotic macule	Relatively common; usually solitary; if multiple consider Peutz–Jeghers syndrome; responds well to cryotherapy or excision
Solar lentigo	Tan coloured; on sun-exposed sites; may closely resemble lentigo maligna; biopsy may be required to distinguish these
Spitz naevus	Red-brown tumour occurring mainly in children; dome-shaped, more vascular than normal naevi; if possible, excise
Halo naevus	Mostly in children, young adults, or women; naevus becomes surrounded by zone of hypopigmentation

Continued

Table 17.1 (*Continued*)

Diagnosis	Clinical features
Seborrhoeic warts/keratoses	Occur in elderly; warty surface; variable pigmentation; usually multiple
Dermatofibroma	Firm pea-like nodule firmly attached to skin; often on limbs of females; may be light brown and itchy
Pyogenic granuloma	Vascular tumour; sudden appearance, often at site of trauma; exophytic; consider possibility of amelanotic melanoma
Basal cell carcinoma	On sun-exposed skin; may be very pigmented; rolled edge; may be ulcerated; can be difficult to distinguish from melanoma
Squamous cell carcinoma	Usually on sun-exposed skin; exophytic tumour; on feet or sun covered skin may mimic amelanotic melanoma
Bowen's disease	Red hyperkeratotic plaque largely on sun-exposed skin; often long history; may develop squamous cell carcinoma
Keratoacanthoma	Rapid onset of dome-shaped nodule on sun exposed skin; may be pigmented; shouldered edge with central keratin plug
Kaposi's sarcoma	Red-brown nodule in skin; in elderly (rare) on legs; in younger age groups on face, palate, trunk in association with AIDS
Benign haemangiomas	Often longstanding vascular nodules usually asymptomatic; often blanch with pressure;
Angiokeratoma	Benign vascular red-brown plaque, occurring from young age; may change colour from intralesional bleed
Glomus tumour	Small red-brown nodule; painful on pressure; can occur under nail
Black heel	Pin-point haemorrhagic points on heel of athletes; often bilateral; history of recent sporting activity
Subungual haematoma	Dark area under nail; usually history of trauma; no pigmentation of proximal nailfold; migrates distally
Tattoo formation	May be history of trauma associated with contact with asphalt, metal oxides, graphite

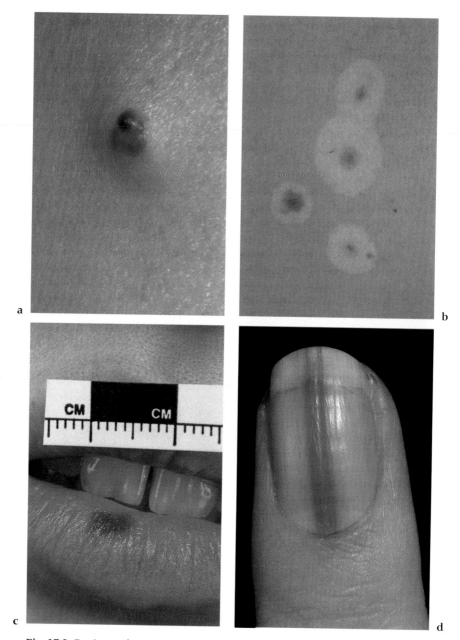

Fig. 17.3 Benign melanocytic lesions. **a**. Blue naevus; **b**. halo naevi; **c**. pigmented labial macule; and **d**. pigmented band of nail.

depth. There is no evidence that such a minor delay adversely affects prognosis.

If regional lymph nodes are palpable, a fine-needle biopsy of these should be carried out to establish if they are infiltrated with tumour; if this is the case, then *en bloc* removal of the regional nodes should be considered, although removal may not significantly alter the overall prognosis.

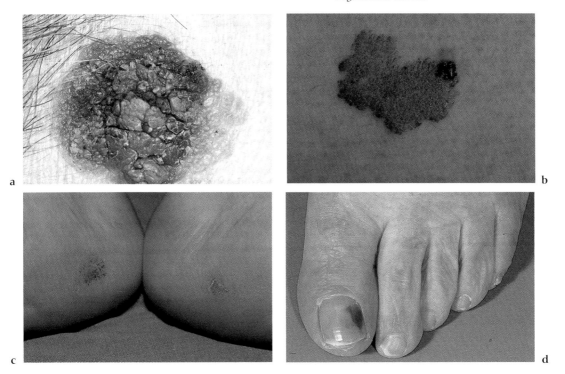

Fig. 17.4 **a**. Pigmented seborrhoeic wart; **b**. haemorrhage within an angiokeratoma; **c**. black heel due to haemorrhage; and **d**. subungual haematoma (note straight proximal margin) which migrates distally.

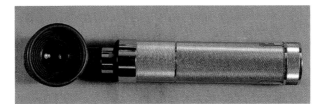

Fig. 17.5 Dermatoscope.

Management of lentigo maligna (melanoma *in situ*)

The risk of a lentigo maligna developing into a lentigo maligna melanoma over the lifetime of the average patient has been estimated at around 30%. Once a lentigo maligna melanoma has developed, the prognosis is similar to that of any other form of melanoma of similar Breslow thickness.

Our view is that formal excision is the treatment of choice for a lentigo maligna, with cryotherapy being reserved for lesions or patients who are not suitable for surgery. Destructive methods of treatment, such as cryotherapy, have disadvantages which include possible failure to treat deep periadenexial melanocytes, inability to detect atypical melanocytes beyond the clinical margin and lack of an excisional specimen to detect invasive melanoma. When possible, excision of lentigo maligna is advised, and leads to cure rates of about 90%. As atypical melanocytes often extend

Table 17.2 Seven-point checklist for suspected malignant melanoma.

Major signs
Change in shape
Change in size
Change in colour

Minor signs
Inflammation
Crusting or bleeding
Sensory change including itch
Diameter ⩾ 7 mm

One or more major signs: consider melanoma
Additional presence of one or more minor signs:
    increased risk of melanoma
Three or four minor signs without major sign: consider
    melanoma

beyond the clinical area of pigmentation, there may be recurrence (Fig. 17.6) and it is therefore advisable, where cosmetically possible, to include a surgical margin of 0.5 cm apparently normal skin, in an attempt to reduce this.

Cryosurgery is an alternative treatment for lentigo maligna, especially in the elderly, who may not be suitable for surgery. However, the recurrence rate seems higher in those who have had cryotherapy (Fig. 17.7) and, without excision of the lesion with formal histopathology, it is impossible to be sure that microinvasion has not occurred in a lentigo maligna, thus making it a true invasive melanoma. If cryosurgery is employed then two freeze–thaw cycles, each of 45–60 s duration, and extending 1 cm beyond

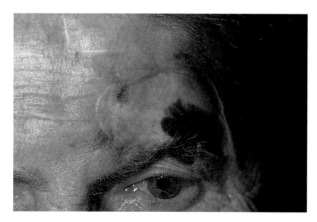

Fig. 17.6 Recurrent melanoma in lentigo maligna treated by excision and grafting.

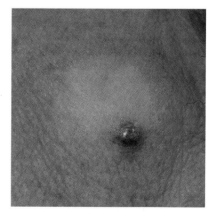

Fig. 17.7 Recurrent nodular melanoma occurring within lentigo maligna treated with cryotherapy. (Courtesy of Dr E.A. Bingham, Royal Victoria Hospital, Belfast.)

the margins of the lesion, are required (see Chapter 12). Freezing should achieve lethal temperatures ($-40°C$ to $-50°C$) in treated tissue as judged by a thermocouple. If pigmentation does develop in an area previously treated with cryotherapy, then a biopsy is mandatory to distinguish between recurrence or reactive lentiginous pigmentation.

Radiotherapy has been used for the treatment of lentigo maligna, with cure rates of 80–90% being reported, but lack of adequate treatment for focal microinvasion can be a problem. Very variable results have been found with the use of 20% topical azelaic acid. These treatments should probably be restricted to frail elderly patients who are unable to undergo other forms of therapy.

17.3 Diagnostic histopathology of melanoma

It is usually fairly easy to distinguish malignant melanoma from the other causes of pigmented lesions on the skin using conventional histopathology. However, the differentiation of a benign but severely dysplastic naevus from a malignant melanoma requires the skills of an experienced skin pathologist. The use of immunocytochemical markers including S100, neurone-specific enolase, anti-human melanoma antibodies (225.28S) and HMB-45 can sometimes be helpful in distinguishing melanomas from other neoplasms. It is generally better to wait the necessary 24 h for conventional

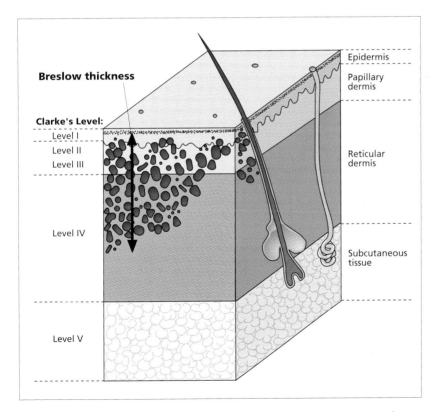

Fig. 17.8 Schematic diagram illustrating assessment of Breslow thickness and Clarke's level of invasion.

wax slides to be processed rather than to insist on an earlier diagnosis based on frozen section specimens, as the latter technique results in artefacts, making the histological diagnosis more difficult.

Essential information to be obtained from the pathologist will include the margins of excision, the type of melanoma, the depth of invasion as assessed by both Breslow thickness and Clarke's level of invasion, the mitotic rate within the tumour and some assessment as to involvement of blood vessels or lymphatic channels. Perhaps the most important of these parameters is the Breslow thickness, which is a measurement of the depth of invasion of melanoma cells, as measured using an ocular micrometer, from the granular layer of the epidermis to the lowest identifiable melanoma cell (Fig. 17.8). This figure is expressed in millimetres of invasion, and is generally accepted to be inversely proportional to the survival rate for melanoma. The Clarke's level of invasion, which records depth of invasion in relation to the structure of the skin (Fig. 17.8) is also useful, as a lesion with a low Breslow thickness but which has invaded as deep as the subcutaneous fat may have a greater degree of metastatic potential than would be apparent from the Breslow thickness alone. Other prognostic features, such as a high mitotic rate, ulceration and tumour cells in and around blood vessels, also suggest a poor prognosis. However, they are more difficult to quantify, and while they may be of use in the management of individual patients, they are less definable for the purposes of research and controlled trials for the treatment of melanoma.

17.4 Staging of melanoma and preoperative assessment

The clinical staging of malignant melanoma (Table 17.3) in conjunction with the Breslow thickness and Clarke's level of tumour invasion enable the planning of definitive further surgery. A thorough history and complete physical examination are usually sufficient to exclude or identify distant metastasis common to sites such as bone and brain. The patient's skin should be fully inspected for other primary melanomas, and for evidence of the dysplastic naevus syndrome, as well as for distant metastases. Regional lymph nodes, liver and spleen should be carefully palpated. Routine investigations are not usually helpful, but it is probably wise to have base-line liver function tests and a chest X-ray. In addition, some authorities advocate a routine liver ultrasound.

Table 17.3 Clinical staging of melanoma.

Clinical stage	Tumour involvement	Prognosis (10-year survival) (%)
Stage I	Local tumour	81
Stage II	Involvement of local lymph nodes	47
Stage III	Disseminated disease	0

17.5 Surgical resection of the primary melanoma

The issue of the optimal margins and depth of excision of melanoma lesions remains the subject of considerable controversy. Definitive guidelines await the results of World Health Organization randomised studies. The rationale for 'wide and deep' resection has been that microsatellites of tumour may be present in the surrounding skin which, if not resected, will lead to both local and distant metastasis. In the past this has resulted in wide local excision with 5 cm margins in all directions, often also including local lymph node resection. However, data from the World Health Organization Melanoma Group and The National Institutes of Health Consensus Development Panel on Early Melanoma suggest that narrower limits, as shown in Table 17.4, do not adversely affect prognosis and are preferable.

In some cases, particularly those involving melanoma on the head and neck, the limits of excision may have to be less than these for the preservation of vital structures; decisions have to be made on the individual circumstances. Some have advocated the use of Mohs' micrographic surgery (see Chapter 20), but this is controversial because it is impossible to totally exclude the presence of melanoma cells on histological slides even with the aid of immunohistochemistry. Melanoma of digits sometimes requires amputation, but functional considerations may make a lesser margin more attractive. On the ear even conservative excision can be disfiguring, although with the development of advanced prosthetic devices a satisfactory cosmetic result is usually achieved.

The issue of depth of excision has also been the subject of much controversy. Until recently, it was suggested that the depth of incision should at least include the superficial fascia. This has now been challenged; many would advocate excision down to the level of fascia, with resection of fascia not being required unless it is infiltrated by tumour. In most cases, the primary defect can be closed directly, but where this is not possible a full thickness skin graft or skin flap may be required. There is no evidence that such closures decrease the detection of local recurrences.

Table 17.4 Resection margins for stage I cutaneous melanoma.

Tumour thickness or site	Surgical margin of normal skin
Melanoma *in situ*	0.5 cm
Melanoma <1.0 mm	1.0 cm
Melanoma ≥1.0 mm, <2 mm	1.0–3.0 cm
Melanoma >2 mm	Not known; 3.0 cm seems prudent
Lentigo maligna melanoma	Base on tumour thickness if feasible; 0.5–1.0 cm margins are usually adequate
Acral and subungual melanoma	Base on tumour thickness if feasible; if surgically difficult, disarticulation of joint proximal to tumour; but consider individual circumstances

17.6 Regional lymph node dissection

The rationale for prophylactic regional lymph node dissection has been the theory that melanoma will metastasise first to the regional lymph nodes, and that the removal of occult node metastasis should improve prognosis. This is another area of controversy. Most European centres have abandoned elective lymph node dissection in favour of close follow up and removal of nodes when they become palpable, while in the USA node dissection is often undertaken for intermediate thickness melanoma whether or not nodes are palpable. It has been shown that lymph node dissection confers no extra benefit in terms of prognosis for patients with melanoma of less than 0.75 mm or more than 4 mm in thickness. There is some evidence that elective lymph node dissection improves survival for lesions in the range of 1.5–3.5 mm in thickness, but it seems that only 15% of patients in this group will benefit from lymph node dissection, and the benefit does not become significant until some 10 years postoperatively. The possible benefit has to be compared with the adverse psychological and cosmetic consequences of mutilating surgery. Further difficulty arises at sites such as the midline, head, neck or upper and lower trunk, where bilateral lymphatic drainage may exist; dye lymphography may help in centres where this is available.

Lymph node dissection can usually be recommended when clinically suspicious regional nodes are identified. Nodal resection may be indicated as a palliative procedure even in the presence of distant metastasis, as ulceration or obstruction of local nodes are often distressing to the patient. When regional nodes are palpable, sampling by needle or incisional biopsy should be carried out.

17.7 Isolated limb perfusion

Despite the fact that isolated limb perfusion has been in use for some 30 years, it remains a controversial treatment for melanoma of the extremities. While it may certainly be helpful in the treatment of regionally recurrent disease, there is no consensus as to its use as a prophylactic measure in patients deemed to be at a high risk of local or distant metastasis at the time of diagnosis of the primary melanoma. A trial of elective limb perfusion is presently being undertaken in the prevention of metastasis in limb melanomas greater than 1.5 mm in thickness.

Limb perfusion can be carried out in two ways.

1 The limb is usually perfused for 1 h with a high concentration of melphalan, administered via a perfusion pump and an extracorporeal circulator, at a temperature of around 40°C. The hyperthermia increases the cytotoxicity of melphalan, thus reducing the total dose that needs to be administered.

2 Alternatively, transient limb perfusion may be used, in which chemotherapy is administered to a limb by intra-arterial infusion following the proximal application of a tourniquet. Although this is a simpler technique, drug levels achieved may not be as high.

Both techniques are often combined with block dissection of the inguinal or obturator lymph node groups, and are usually used for 'limb salvage' when dealing with thick melanomas. Side effects of isolated limb perfusion include pain, nerve damage, arterial and venous thrombosis, limb oedema, loss of the limb and up to 2% mortality. These techniques are not widely available and should only be performed in institutions with special expertise in their use.

17.8 Follow up

The patient should be instructed regarding screening for new pigmented lesions, changes in pre-existing naevi and sun protection. Where dysplastic naevus syndrome is deemed to be present, family screening may also be considered for first-degree relatives of the patient. The follow up of a patient following the excision of a melanoma is dictated by an assessment of the individual's risk of developing either a recurrence or a second primary melanoma. It is suggested that follow up should be monthly for the first 3 months, 3-monthly thereafter up to 2 years, then 6-monthly for 5 years, followed by an annual review.

At follow up, the surgical scar should be checked for signs of local recurrence, and the regional lymph nodes, liver and spleen should be palpated. Patients should have a total body skin examination for any evidence of new primary melanomas, as the chance of a person developing a second primary is approximately 4%. They should be questioned regarding symptoms which might indicate bone or brain metastasis. An annual chest X-ray is recommended by some for patients with primary tumours greater than 1.5 mm in thickness, but routine laboratory tests are not considered useful.

17.9 Prognosis

The prognosis of patients with melanoma depends largely on the depth of invasion of tumour as assessed by both Breslow and Clarke's thickness (Table 17.5); the presence of gross or microscopic ulceration worsens prognosis, as does the presence of satellite lesions.

The prognosis is also adversely affected by increasing age, male sex and for primary lesions on the trunk. It is now generally accepted that pregnancy is not an adverse factor for melanoma and the diagnosis of melanoma in pregnancy is not sufficient medical justification for termination of pregnancy. The prognosis of women who have had a thin melanoma excised during pregnancy is unchanged. Women who have had a thick melanoma (greater than 2 mm) are probably best advised to postpone pregnancy for 2–3 years as recurrence is most likely during this period, and patients with advanced melanoma may not survive to raise their

Table 17.5 Prognosis of cutaneous melanoma based on tumour thickness.

Risk category	Melanoma thickness (mm)	5-year survival (%)
Low	<0.76	96–99
Low	0.76–1.50	87–94
Intermediate	1.51–4.00	66–77
High	>4.00	<50

family. There appears to be no evidence that the use of oral contraceptives or hormone replacement therapy has any adverse effect on the prognosis of melanoma.

17.10 Treatment of advanced melanoma

Surgery for advanced metastatic disease has a place in the reduction of tumour load and in the palliation of isolated metastases in the brain, lung or gastrointestinal tract. In addition, radiotherapy can achieve good palliation with reduction of bone pain, diminution of cerebral metastases and control of large soft tissue metastases which might otherwise ulcerate and bleed. Radiotherapy is, however, unlikely to influence the long-term outcome of secondary metastasis. Chemotherapy has a role in advanced disease, but the results are not spectacular. The two drugs presently felt to be most effective against melanoma are dacarbazine and vindesine; a combination of these two drugs can be used to reduce the overall toxicity while increasing the quality of life and duration of response. Other multiple drug combinations have been advocated, including the use of carmustine, cisplatin, tamoxifen and bleomycin, and result in remission in 40–50% of cases, which although often only partial and short-lived, has lasted for several years in some cases. More recent drugs, of unproven efficacy as yet, such as fotemustine and mitozolamide, are under investigation. Regimens using interferon, interleukins and lymphokine-activated killer cells, combined with cytotoxic agents, are also undergoing assessment. Management of advanced metastatic disease is best undertaken in specialist centres with considerable experience of these drug combinations. Even in experienced hands, response is only likely to continue beyond 1 year in a small proportion of patients.

Bibliography

Ackerman AB. What nevus is dysplastic, a syndrome and the commonest precursor of malignant melanoma? A riddle and an answer. *Histopathology* 1988; 13: 241–56.

Austoker J. Melanoma: prevention and early diagnosis. *Br Med J* 1994; 308: 1682–6.

Balch CM. The role of elective lymph node dissection of melanoma: rationale, results and controversies. *J Clin Oncol* 1988; 6: 163–72.

Clark WH Jr, Elder DE, Guerry D 4th, Epstein MN, Greene MH, Van-Horn M. A study of tumor progression: the precursor lesions of superficial spreading and nodular melanoma. *Hum Pathol* 1984; 15: 1147–65.

Cohen LM. Lentigo maligna and lentigo maligna melanoma. *J Am Acad Dermatol* 1995; 33: 923–36.

Cohen PJ, Lambert WC, Hill G, Schwartz RA. Melanoma. In: Schwartz RA, ed. *Skin Cancer; Recognition and Management*. New York: Springer-Verlag, 1988; 99–140.

Evans RD, Kopf AW, Lew RA *et al*. Risk factors for the development of malignant melanoma-I: review of case-control studies. *J Dermatol Surg Oncol* 1988; 14: 393–408.

Gari LM, Rivers JK, Kopf AW. Melanomas arising in large congenital nevocytic nevi: a prospective study. *Pediatr Dermatol* 1988; 5: 151–8.

Ghussen F, Kruger I, Groth W, Stutzer H. The role of regional hyperthermic cytostatic perfusion in the treatment of extremity melanoma. *Cancer* 1988; 61: 654–9.

Green A, Siskind V, Hansen ME, Hanson L, Leech P. Melanocytic nevi in school-children in Queensland. *J Am Acad Dermatol* 1989; 20: 1054–60.

Handfield-Jones SE, Smith NP. Malignant melanoma in childhood. *Br J Dermatol* 1996; 134: 607–16.

Ho VC, Sober AJ. Therapy for cutaneous melanoma: an update. *J Am Acad Dermatol* 1990; 22: 159–76.

Jatoi I, Gore ME. Sex, pregnancy, hormones and melanoma. *Br Med J* 1993; 307: 2–3.

Koh HK, Michalik E, Sober AJ *et al.* Lentigo maligna melanoma has no better prognosis than other types of melanoma. *J Clin Oncol* 1984; 2: 994–1001.

Lees VC, Briggs JC. Effect of initial biopsy procedure on prognosis in stage I invasive cutaneous malignant melanoma. *Br J Plast Surg* 1991; 78: 1108–10.

Lyons JH, Cockerell CJ. Elective lymph node dissection for melanoma. *J Am Acad Dermatol* 1994; 30: 467–80.

MacKie RM. Malignant melanoma. In: MacKie RM (ed.) *Skin Cancer.* London: Martin Dunitz, 1989: 178–201.

MacKie RM, Hole DJ. Incidence and thickness of primary tumours and survival of patients with cutaneous malignant melanoma in relation to socioeconomic status. *Br Med J* 1996; 312: 1125–8.

Malone ME, Jones DB, Sexton FM. Pigmented basal cell carcinoma: investigation of 70 cases. *J Am Acad Dermatol* 1992; 27: 74–8.

Nachbar F, Stolz W, Merkle T *et al.* The ABCD rule of dermatoscopy. *J Am Acad Dermatol* 1994; 30: 551–9.

Nakajima T, Watanabe S, Sato Y, Kameya T, Shimosato Y, Ishihara K. Immunohistochemical demonstration of S-100 protein in malignant melanoma and pigmented nevus, and its diagnostic application. *Cancer* 1982; 50: 912–18.

Rigel DS, Rivers JK, Kopf AW *et al.* Dysplastic nevi. Markers for increased risk for melanoma. *Cancer* 1989; 63: 386–9.

Seraly MP, Rhodes AR. Surgical margins and elective lymph node dissection in the management of localised primary cutaneous melanoma. In: Dahl MV, Lynch PJ, eds. *Current Opinion in Dermatology.* Philadelphia: Current Science, 1993: 53–8.

Slue W, Kopf AW, Rivers JK. Total body photographs of dysplastic nevi. *Arch Dermatol* 1988; 124: 1239–43.

Stolz W, Braun-Falco O, Bilek P *et al. Colour Atlas of Dermatoscopy.* Berlin: Blackwell Wissenschafts-Verlag GmbH, 1993.

Timmons MJ. Malignant melanoma excision margins: plastic surgery audit in Britain and Ireland, 1991, and a review. *Br J Plast Surg* 1993; 46: 525–31.

Travers RL, Sober AJ, Berwick M *et al.* Increased thickness of pregnancy-associated melanoma. *Br J Dermatol* 1995; 132: 876–83.

Veronesi U, Cascinelli N, Adamus J *et al.* Thin stage of primary cutaneous melanoma: comparison of excision with margins of one or three centimeters. *N Engl J Med* 1988; 318: 1159–62.

18 Nail surgery

18.1 Anatomy of the nail apparatus

The nail plate is produced from the matrix which extends some 6 mm proximal to the proximal nail fold forwards to appear in some digits as the greyish white semi-circular lunula, which is the visible portion of the matrix underlying the nail plate (Fig. 18.1a). The nail matrix has a firm attachment to its underlying papillary dermis, being anchored by a number of basal cell projections or anchoring filaments. The matrix epithelium consists of basal cells, the onychocytes, which undergo keratinisation to form the nail plate. The upper surface of the nail plate is derived from the proximal matrix, while the deeper portion is derived from the distal part of the nail matrix. Melanocytes occur abundantly in the nail matrix of black people, but less frequently in Oriental or Caucasian people. Longitudinal bands of pigmentation in the plate are the result of foci of melanocytes in the matrix. The nail plate, commonly referred to as the nail, is the result of keratinisation in the matrix, and grows distally while being held firmly adherent to the underlying nail bed.

The nail bed consists of an epithelium, with longitudinally aligned epidermal ridges, which in turn is attached to its dermis. The epithelial cells of the nail bed are slowly proliferating stratified cells with little tendency to keratinisation. The nail bed dermis is highly vascular and contains glomus organs. Distal to the nail bed is the hyponychium; the extension of the finger epidermis ends in the distal groove, which is the point at which the nail bed finally separates from the underlying tissue (Fig. 18.1b). The nail cuticle appears proximally under the proximal nail fold and is an extension of the proximal nail fold skin onto the surface of the nail plate, where it continues for a short distance before being shed. The cuticle arises as a result of orthokeratinisation of the distal portion of the proximal nail fold, and serves to seal the potential space between the nail plate and the proximal nail fold.

The nail plate emerges from under the proximal nail fold at an angle to the surface of the dorsal digital skin which should not be less than 180° (Lovibond's angle). On either side of each nail are the nail grooves, which are bounded by the two lateral nail folds.

The nail apparatus is held in place by dense sclerotic mesenchyme underneath the nail unit, which anchors it to the periosteum. The underlying phalanx thus has a role in determining the shape and convexity of the nail, and the nail in turn serves to protect the distal digit. Fingernails grow faster than toenails; fingernails growing at a rate of 0.1 mm/day, while toenails grow around one-half to one-third as quickly.

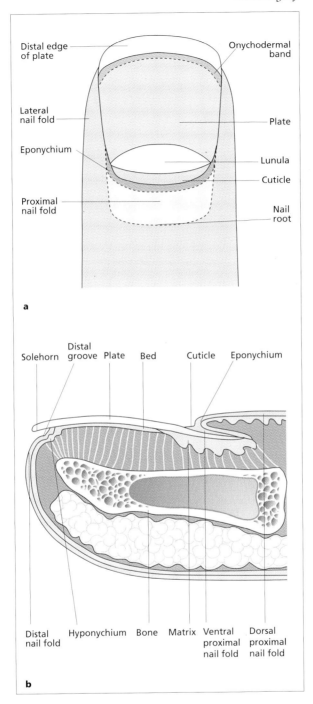

Fig. 18.1 Anatomy of the nail unit: **a**. Dorsal view and **b**. sagittal view.

18.2 General aspects of nail surgery

Anaesthesia can be performed by either a digital nerve block, as described in Chapter 5, or simply by anaesthetising the nail unit using the distal 'wing block' (Fig. 18.2). This is useful for surgery on the nail folds, matrix and proximal nail bed. The injection entry site should be about 3 mm proximal

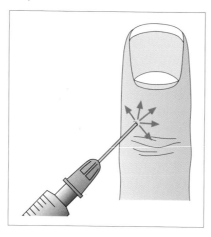

Fig. 18.2 Wing block digital anaesthesia in the region of the proximal nail fold.

to the junction of the proximal nail fold and lateral nail folds. The needle is advanced distally and downwards to introduce anaesthetic along the base of the phalanx, thereby anaesthetising the terminal branches of the lateral digital nerve. Less than 0.5 ml of 1% lignocaine is usually required on each side. The injection can be continued in the region of the proximal nail fold. It may be necessary to use a supplementary distal injection for more distal procedures. Where considerable postoperative pain is anticipated, mixing a short-acting anaesthetic, such as lignocaine, with a long-acting anaesthetic, such as bupivacaine, may result in decreased postoperative pain.

Application of a sterile surgical glove, from which the relevant fingertip has been removed, to the hand being operated upon, provides a sterile surgical field. Rolling the glove finger proximally to the base of the digit may produce an effective tourniquet (glove tourniquet).

All patients who have had hand or foot surgery should have their limb elevated as much as possible for 48 h to reduce postoperative oedema and pain. Pain following surgery to the nail apparatus can be severe, such that the patient will usually require a combination of paracetamol and codeine (Paracodol®, Co-codamol®, Kapake®) or a non-steroidal anti-inflammatory agent.

The dressing of a nail following surgery should be sufficiently absorbent to collect any oozing blood or serosanguineous fluid, but must not be so tight as to compromise the circulation, especially in the setting of potential postoperative oedema. It is usually best to start the dressing with either paraffin gauze or a haemostat such as gelatin foam (Gelfoam®) or calcium alginate (Kaltostat®). The nail is then wrapped in gauze which can be secured in place using Tubinette® or adhesive tape. It is imperative that the dressing is not too tight and takes account of the possibility of postoperative swelling. Ideally, the dressing should be changed daily for the first few days. The nail unit should be carefully washed in 3% hydrogen peroxide, before a topical antibiotic is applied and the area is redressed.

18.3 Achieving a bloodless field

Many nail surgery procedures, such as matricectomy or nail bed surgery,

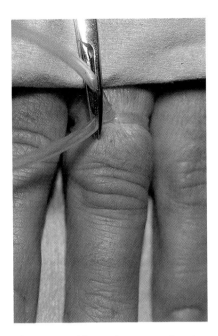

Fig. 18.3 Rubber catheter tourniquet
secured around digit with a haemostat.

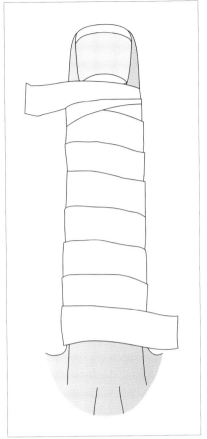

Fig. 18.4 Exsanguination of digit using
a Penrose drain wrapped around digit.

necessitate a bloodless field. One approach is to use a glove tourniquet, a
rubber catheter tourniquet secured with a haemostat (Fig. 18.3) or a rubber
band tourniquet, where loops of a rubber band, doubled or tripled over the
base of a finger, are tightened by means of winding a haemostat placed
between the loops. Alternatively, the digit may first be exsanguinated by
applying a Penrose drain, wrapped tightly around the digit in overlapping
loops starting distally (Fig. 18.4) in such a way as to effectively 'milk' the
blood from the distal digit. A separate drain is then wrapped around the
base of the digit and tightened firmly by twisting the separate ends before
application of a haemostat. The distal drain is then removed leaving a dry
surgical field. The time at which the proximal tourniquet is applied should
be noted, as it is prudent not to leave this on longer than 20 min, or
10–15 min in those with a history of vascular disease or diabetes.

18.4 Subungual haematoma

One of the most frequent indications for surgical intervention on the nail is the development of a subungual haematoma. This usually occurs as a result of blunt trauma to the nail, and is associated with severe pain which can be relieved, if necessary, by release of the haematoma. The history of trauma helps to distinguish a subungual haematoma from the more sinister subungual melanoma.

Most subungual haematomas do not require treatment, being resorbed on their own. If the haematoma is painful, it can be drained by application of the end of an opened paper clip (which has been heated over a spirit lamp) to the area, which makes a hole in the nail through which the subungual haematoma may be evacuated. An alternative is the battery-operated Aaron® nail drill, which comes with disposable, sterile drill bits and is convenient to use.

If the haematoma involves over 25% of the nail bed area this may indicate a more serious injury requiring removal of the nail plate and formal repair of the nail bed. X-rays should be performed to exclude the possibility of a fracture of the underlying phalanx. Repair of the nail bed can be carried out by preparing the patient as for nail bed biopsy (see below) and suturing the torn nail bed with a 6/0 absorbable suture.

18.5 Treatment of ingrowing toenails

Ingrowing toenails mostly involve the great toe, and are often caused by the patient cutting back or tearing the lateral border of the distal nail plate, allowing spicules of the nail plate to be inserted into the lateral nail fold. This process is exacerbated by the wearing of tight shoes.

For the earliest symptoms of pain, swelling and redness of the lateral nail fold, conservative treatment may often obviate the need for formal nail surgery. The lateral, distal nail plate margin is extracted from the skin and cotton wool, which has been soaked in antiseptic, is worked in under the lateral nail edge and between it and the lateral sulcus. This approach usually relieves the pain and inflammation quickly and can be carried out, until symptoms subside, by the patient at home.

If the problem becomes more persistent, then surgery will probably be required. This usually involves a lateral nail plate excision and phenolisation of the appropriate area of the nail matrix. The area is anaesthetised, and the digit is exsanguinated and has a tourniquet applied as described above. The nail plate is split longitudinally at its lateral one-fifth using either a nail splitter or a No. 10 scalpel blade. This lateral nail strip can then be freed by grasping its distal portion using an artery forceps, and rotating it towards the rest of the nail, such that the lateral border of the nail is elevated first, minimising the risk of leaving nail spicules in the lateral groove (Fig. 18.5a). The lateral nail fold sulcus can then be curetted to remove any residual spicules of nail. The lateral portion of the nail matrix is next treated with liquified phenol (80%) soaked onto a small cotton bud, which is pushed as proximally as possible into the defect between the lateral and proximal nail fold. The normal skin around the proximal and lateral nail fold can be protected by a layer of Vaseline® to avoid phenol burns in this area. The phenol should be applied not only to the matrix but also along the lateral sulcus for some 3 min, before being neutralised by irrigation with

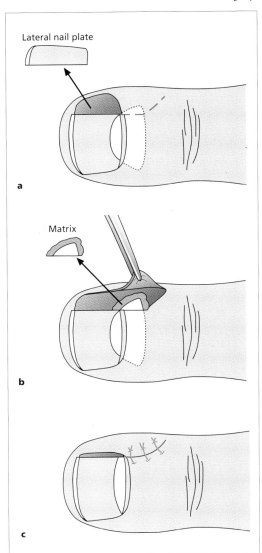

Fig. 18.5 Wedge excision of ingrowing toenail.
a. Removal of lateral nail plate; **b**. removal of matrix; and **c**. suturing of proximal nail fold.

normal saline. Using this technique, recurrence rates of less than 10% in the first postoperative year have been achieved.

An alternative approach involves surgical excision of the lateral nail matrix. After removal of the nail strip, a green needle is inserted along the lateral groove until it touches bone; this helps to identify the lateral horn of the nail matrix, which usually lies more posteriorly and laterally than expected. An incision is then made in the proximal nail fold region which arcs proximally and laterally to expose the lateral matrix (Fig. 18.5b) region, and the matrix is then removed from the area around the needle by excision and curettage before the proximal nail fold is sutured (Fig. 18.5c). Where there is marked hypertrophy of the lateral nail fold, then the involved skin may be excised distally.

If desired, the lateral nail fold can be sutured back to the nail plate using 2/3 non-absorbable sutures which pass through the nail plate and the lateral nail fold. Placement of these sutures can be facilitated by first making holes in the nail using a needle. The digit is then dressed with a topical antibiotic and a digit dressing, as described above. Where there is marked infection of an ingrowing toenail, it is wise to cover the procedure with a course of a systemic antibiotic.

18.6 Nail plate avulsion with or without permanent matricectomy

Removal of the nail plate with matricectomy, which leads to permanent destruction of the nail matrix and prevention of nail growth, can be used in the treatment of ingrowing toenails, pincer nail syndrome, difficult cases of onychomycosis, onychogryphosis or other chronic symptomatic nail conditions. Nail plate avulsion on its own without matricectomy can be used to permit exploration of the nail bed or nail matrix zones. After achieving anaesthesia and a bloodless field, the distal nail plate can be separated from the nail bed using a Freer nasal septal elevator or blunt artery forceps; the latter is more likely to damage the nail bed (Fig. 18.6). The nail plate should be easily cleaved from the nail bed, although there will be some resistance to advancement of blunt dissection until the nail matrix area is reached, when a characteristic 'give' is felt; at this point, blunt dissection can be stopped. The sides of the digit are then held firmly while the nail plate is rocked from side to side to loosen it from the matrix and the underlying bed. The elevator is next inserted under the cuticle at the proximal nail fold to loosen the dorsal attachments. The nail plate can now be

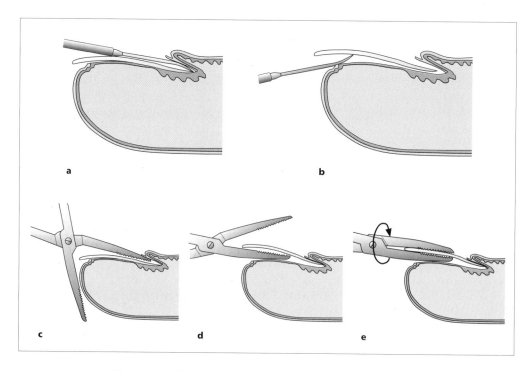

a

b

c

d

e

Fig. 18.6 Avulsion of nail plate using: (**a, b**) Freer nasal septal elevator; and (**c–e**) blunt artery forceps

removed quite easily by grasping the plate distally with an artery forceps, and pulling distally while exerting a rocking movement until the nail plate comes free.

If a permanent matricectomy is required, the matrix can be exposed by cutting back into the proximal nail fold region, incising at the junctions of the lateral and proximal nail folds on each side, and reflecting the proximal nail fold back. The latter can be held back using skin hooks to fully expose the nail matrix area. The matrix can then be ablated by firmly applying phenol (80%)-saturated cotton buds directly onto it for approximately 3 min. It is important that the phenol be applied to the entire matrix, including the area of the lunula, under the proximal nail fold and both lateral nail horns. Following phenolisation, the area should be flooded with saline or 70% alcohol to neutralise the phenol, before the proximal nail fold is sutured back into place.

If bleeding persists following release of the tourniquet, the area can be packed with a calcium alginate dressing followed by a dressing to the digit. Healing will occur, with the nail bed taking on the thickened leathery appearance of a pseudo-nail.

This procedure for nail matrix phenolisation described above has a relatively good rate of success, but a recent study has shown that a combination of curettage and subsequent phenol application results in almost 100% eradication of the matrix.

An alternative to chemical matricectomy is surgical resection of the matrix area. This can be used in patients with advanced vascular disease involving the digit, when chemical phenolisation is relatively contra-indicated. The matrix is exposed as before, and the nail matrix excised down to, and including, the periosteum; this usually results in total ablation of the nail apparatus. Some surgeons prefer to resect not only the matrix area but also the rest of the nail bed, prior to application of a split skin graft or free nail bed graft to the area as, in some patients, nail-forming tissue is not confined to the matrix area.

18.7 Biopsy of the nail unit

Biopsy of various parts of the nail unit is often required for either diagnostic or therapeutic purposes. The nail matrix may be biopsied in the case of pigmented nail streaks to exclude the possibility of a malignant melanoma, or for diagnostic purposes in dystrophic nails such as in lichen planus or psoriasis, or for the removal of any tumour arising in the matrix area.

Nail bed biopsies can be used to diagnose and treat Bowen's disease, squamous cell carcinoma, melanoma, glomus tumours or other tumours of the nail bed. Squamous cell carcinoma of the nail should be considered in any papillomatous growth, persistent erosion, fissure or hyperkeratotic lesion of the nail folds. Patients should always be warned about the possibility of permanent nail dystrophy following biopsy.

The biopsy technique sometimes referred to as longitudinal resection *en bloc*, which includes the nail fold, matrix and bed (Fig. 18.7), is useful in determining and defining disease processes such as psoriasis and lichen planus, although it probably has most place in research studies.

Nail matrix biopsy

Anaesthesia is induced by a ring block of the digit, and the digit is exsanguinated as previously described. Incisions are made from the angle at the junction of the proximal and lateral nail fold proximally, to make the proximal nail fold region into a small flap which can be retracted proximally (Fig. 18.8a). The nail plate should not be disturbed before biopsy of the matrix, as it tends to fix the matrix in position, allowing better visualisation. It may, however, be necessary to avulse part or all of the nail plate when a pigmented lesion extends distally beyond the lunula or onto the nail bed, to exclude the possibility of melanoma. There are several techniques for taking a biopsy of the nail matrix but whichever method is used it is best, if possible, to take the biopsy from the distal segment of the matrix since this avoids subsequent nail dystrophy or nail splitting.

Fortunately, pigmented lesions usually lie in the distal segment of the matrix, allowing the proximal part of the matrix, which forms the surface of the nail plate, to be left undisturbed. The nail matrix biopsy can be taken as a small punch (Fig. 18.8a) or, if necessary, a transverse fusiform biopsy can be performed in the anterior zone (Fig. 18.8b). It is generally not necessary to suture these matrix defects, especially if they are kept below 3–4 mm in diameter.

Occasionally, it may be necessary to take a longitudinal fusiform biopsy through the entire length of the matrix (Fig. 18.8c). The biopsy specimen taken should be incised all the way down to bone. This does increase the risk of dystrophy to the nail, especially if it is greater than 3 mm in diameter, and it is best to try and close the defect with absorbable sutures to prevent

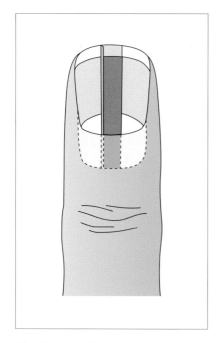

Fig. 18.7 Longitudinal nail resection *en bloc.*

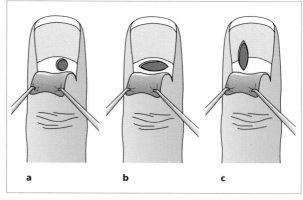

Fig. 18.8 Nail matrix biopsy. **a.** Reflection of proximal nail fold and punch biopsy; **b.** fusiform nail matrix biopsy; **c.** longitudinal fusiform biopsy through entire length of matrix.

permanent longitudinal nail dystrophy. This can be done with a fine 6/0 vicryl suture, but a special suture material termed 6/0 surgical plain gut type A (Ethilon®) is available, which is absorbed very quickly and helps to reduce the possibility of nail dystrophy.

After the biopsy has been performed the proximal nail fold should be sutured back into place, along the lines of incision.

A similar approach may be used to excise tumours in the region of the proximal nail fold (Fig. 18.9).

Nail bed biopsy

Nail bed biopsies can be taken either with the nail plate being left largely intact or after the nail plate has been partially or completely removed. It is possible to perform a biopsy of the nail bed for diagnostic purposes, say in

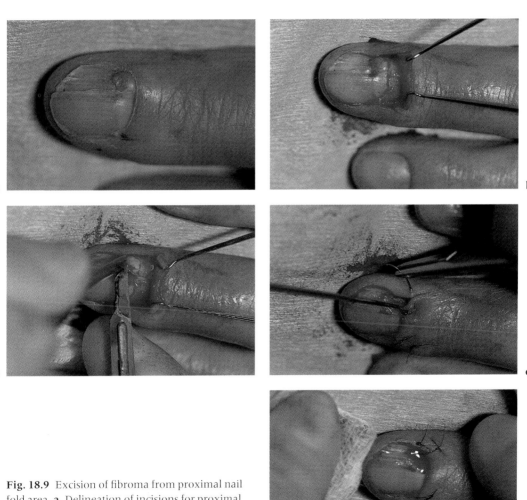

a

b

c

d

e

Fig. 18.9 Excision of fibroma from proximal nail fold area. **a**. Delineation of incisions for proximal nail fold reflection; **b**. proximal nail fold reflected; **c**. excision of tumour; **d**. suturing of incisions in proximal nail fold; and **e**. excision and closure complete.

the case of Bowen's disease, through the nail plate without removing the plate. After anaesthesia and exsanguination of the digit, a 4-mm punch is used to penetrate the nail plate, and the 4-mm disc of nail plate is removed to allow visualisation of the underlying nail bed (Fig. 18.10a,b). A 3-mm punch is then used to core out a cylinder of the nail bed, taking the biopsy down to bone. The slightly larger diameter nail plate defect allows the biopsy to be dissected free; bleeding will usually stop spontaneously under pressure.

For the diagnosis and treatment of tumours, for example, pigmented lesions on the nail bed or glomus tumours, it is usually better to remove the nail plate. The overlying nail plate can either be avulsed, as described above or, after making bilateral incisions proximally from the junctions of the lateral and proximal nail folds, the nail can be reflected backwards after separation of the nail from the nail bed using Freer's nasal septal elevator. Biopsies of the nail bed should, in contrast to those of the nail matrix, when possible, be longitudinal in direction; they should be limited to a width of less than 3 mm. It is often easier to lift the end of the specimen with a 30-gauge needle before using sharp curved iris scissors to excise the specimen from the periosteum below. Small excision biopsies can be left unsutured but for larger defects the area can be closed using absorbable sutures to the nail bed (Fig. 18.11). If the nail plate has not been avulsed, it can be 'reflected' back onto the nail bed, and the incisions are then sutured. The patient must be informed of the possibility that the nail plate may be shed following operation, as some damage at the nail matrix–plate interface may be caused by the reflection of the nail. However, more often than not the nail plate can be maintained.

18.8 Myxoid cysts

Myxoid cysts are formed as a result of a synovial outpouching of the capsule of the distal interphalangeal joint (Fig. 18.12), and appear at the proximal nail fold as translucent cystic lesions 2–4 mm in diameter. Puncture of these reveals a clear viscous fluid. They may produce longitudinal grooving of the nail by compressing the adjacent nail matrix. The treatment of myxoid cysts can be conservative, with repeated release of the mucoid contents using a sterile needle, with a view to producing sufficient fibrosis to obliterate the lesion. Alternatively, the lesion can be excised, following reflection of the proximal nail fold skin (Fig. 18.13), with a Freer septum elevator being inserted into the proximal nail groove under the lesion to eliminate the risk of damaging the nail matrix or the extensor tendon. The resultant wound may be allowed to heal by secondary intention, and with daily dressings a good result should be achieved in a few weeks. To prevent recurrence, the connection to the underlying joint should be found and tied off. This can be delineated by injecting sterile methylene blue into the distal interphalangeal joint through the palmar aspect of the finger and waiting for the blue dye to appear in the cyst, before progressing to surgery. A blue tract connecting the cyst with the underlying joint may often be visualised in this way in the loose connective tissue between the cyst and the joint.

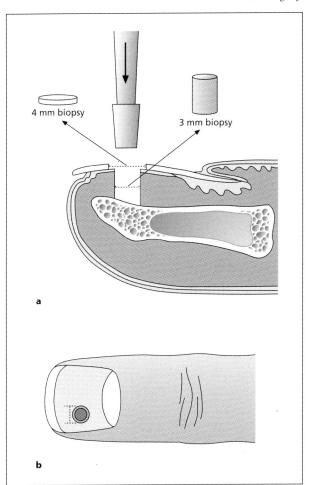

4 mm biopsy

3 mm biopsy

a

b

Fig. 18.10 Nail bed biopsy using the double-punch technique. **a**. Sagittal view and **b**. view from above.

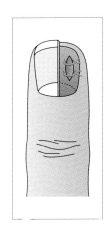

Fig. 18.11 Fusiform biopsy of nail bed after partial nail plate removal.

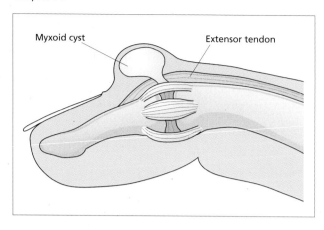

Fig. 18.12 Origin of myxoid cyst.

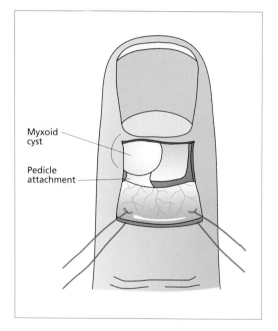

Fig. 18.13 Reflection of proximal nail fold to visualise myxoid cyst.

An alternative treatment of myxoid cysts is the use of cryosurgery. The mucoid contents should first be expressed by pricking the cyst with a sterile needle, after which one 20 s freeze–thaw cycle may be given. If this proves unsuccessful, the treatment may be repeated by using two 30 s freeze–thaw cycles, although this often results in a painful, ulcerated lesion which may take some weeks to heal. Recently, the infrared coagulator (see Chapter 7, Section 7.4) has been used to treat myxoid cysts.

18.9 Urea paste keratolysis

Urea paste can be used as a keratolytic to remove dystrophic nails when, but only when, there is marked subungual hyperkeratosis, especially in the setting of onychomychosis or psoriasis. It is not effective on normal nails.

The nail is first soaked in water for about 20 min, and urea paste is then applied over the surface of the nail and under the distal nail plate. It is held in place using plastic wrap film, such as cling film or an Opsite® dressing, for between 3 and 7 days. If desired, the skin surrounding the nail can be protected with tincture of benzoin, but this is not an absolute requirement. At the end of the period of occlusion, the nail and the subungual hyperkeratosis should have turned white and can be easily dislodged.

The formula for the production of this urea paste is as follows.

- Urea (finely ground powder): 60 g.
- White beeswax: 7.5 g.
- Hydrous lanolin: 30 g.
- White petrolatum: 37 g.
- Silica gel type H: 15 g.

The urea paste is made by melting beeswax at a temperature of 85°C; the other ingredients are added to the beeswax in a stainless steel blender while blending takes place. The resulting paste has a shelf life of 6 months.

Bibliography

Baran R, Dawber RPR (eds). *Diseases of the Nails and their Management*. Oxford: Blackwell Scientific Publications, 1994.

Greig JD, Anderson JH, Ireland AJ, Anderson JR. The surgical treatment of ingrowing toenails. *J Bone Joint Surg* 1991; 73: 131–3.

Kemmett D, Colver GB. Myxoid cysts treated by infra-red coagulation. *Clin Exp Dermatol* 1994; 19: 118–20.

Scher RK. Biopsy of the matrix of a nail. *J Dermatol Surg Oncol* 1980; 6: 19–21.

Scher RK, Daniel CR. *Nails: Therapy, Diagnosis, Surgery*. Philadelphia: WB Saunders, 1990.

Zaias N. *The Nail in Health and Disease*. Connecticut: Appleton & Lange, 1990.

19 Cosmetic and aesthetic procedures

19.1 Telangiectasia and superficial veins

Classification of telangiectasia

Telangiectasia have been characteristically classified into four patterns according to their clinical appearance.

1 Simple linear telangiectasia. Red linear telangiectasia occur especially on the nose or legs and the blue linear form occurs most often on the legs. Those on the face may be associated with chronic alcohol consumption, rosacea or solar damage.

2 Arborising telangiectasia. These occur most commonly on the lower legs of women and should not be confused with groups of dilated superficial veins which occur on the lateral thigh.

3 Spider telangiectasia or spider naevi. These are red and arise from a central filling arteriole; pressure on the central feeding vessel causes blanching of the radiating vessels.

4 Punctiform (papular). These occur most frequently as part of genetic syndromes (e.g. Osler–Rendu–Weber syndrome) or collagen vascular diseases.

Telangiectasia on the face are mostly asymptomatic and requests for treatment are as a result of their cosmetic appearance. Those on the legs, being both of the simple and the arborising type, may become slightly painful before or during the menstrual period. It is also important on the legs to decide if there is a contribution from associated varicose veins, so that incompetent perforating veins can be dealt with before treatment is undertaken for the more superficial small diameter vessels.

19.2 Electrosurgery treatment of telangiectasia

Hyfrecator

For many telangiectasia the use of a Birtcher Hyfrecator® is adequate, with the instrument set at a very low current. The unit can be used in the unipolar mode with the setting as low as possible, adjusting upwards until enough spark is produced to enter the vessel. It is not possible to use local anaesthesia while doing this procedure as this will cause shutdown of the telangiectasia, either on a volume basis or because of vasoconstriction, or as an effect of the anaesthetic.

For small vessels it is usually not necessary to enter the vessel itself, but merely to induce sparking over the vessel by placing the hyfrecator tip about 1 mm above the vascular lesion. For vessels larger than 1 mm in diameter it is best to canalise the vessel with an insulated disposable epilating needle. A special needle adapter is available to attach such needles to the hyfrecator tip.

Whether the vessel is cannulated or the hyfrecator tip is used as an over-lying probe, the current jumps into the vessel rather than going through the skin, as the blood in the vessel is more conductive than the surrounding skin. Most patients accept this form of therapy readily, especially if allowed a brief respite after every 10 bursts of energy. Vessels around the nose and eyes are more painful to treat and those around the columella or ala nasi can induce either sneezing or a tear response. Using this technique, it is only rarely that a tiny scar is seen as a white dot on the skin at the site of entry of current. This is usually not a cosmetic problem, but clearly the patient should be advised about the possibility before undergoing therapy. Scarring tends to be greater on leg vessels, where a line of white dot scars known as the 'string of pearls' can be seen; because of this, other methods may be preferred on this site.

Hyfrecator for spider naevi

Because of the vascularity of the central vessel in the spider naevus, the use of electrosurgery may leave a small white scar. Again, anaesthesia may not be able to be used, depending on the size of the vessel (Fig. 19.1), and the electrosurgical spark should be directed towards the central feeding vessel. Alternatively, for this type of lesion cold point cautery can be used. The spiral peripheral wire heats a central sharp wire which is used to touch the centre of the spider naevus. This, however, also has the disadvantage of possible scarring.

Spider naevi may also be treated with cryosurgery, perhaps best per-formed using a cryoprobe for accurate application, and using no more than a 10 s freeze–thaw cycle.

When the above techniques of ablating spider naevus are not successful and a tunable dye laser is not available, it is possible to remove the central blood vessel feeding the spider using a 2-mm punch, closing the defect using one suture. This has the disadvantage of leaving a permanent scar, although it may be much easier to camouflage than a large spider naevus.

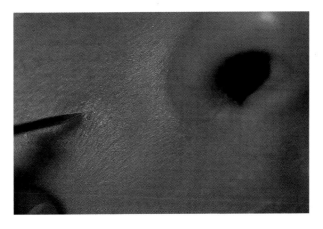

Fig. 19.1 Treatment of spider naevus with hyfrecator.

19.3 Sclerotherapy

Sclerotherapy involves the injection of sclerosant chemicals into blood vessels, such that thrombosis of the blood vessel is achieved, followed by fibrosis and obliteration of the vessel. This is most frequently used for small dilated superficial veins on the lower legs, although of course it can be used for vessels of much larger diameter as for treatment of varicose veins.

Sclerotherapy agents

The sclerosants that are currently available, with their potential side effects, are discussed individually below.

1 Sodium tetradecyl sulphate is a long-chain fatty acid salt with many of the properties of a soap. Initially, it was used as a 1% solution, but this led to a very high rate of superficial necrosis of overlying skin and hyper-pigmentation. The recommended concentration now is that of 0.33%. Systemic reactions including anaphylaxis, generalised urticaria and maculopapular eruptions have been described, and some sclerotherapists suggest a 3-day pre- and post-therapy course of antihistamines.

2 Hypertonic saline can be used at concentrations of 20–23.4% and has a good ability to sclerose arborising telangiectasia. The advantages of this agent are that it has no potential for allergic reactions and it is inexpensive; however, it can cause stinging and burning on injection, as well as muscle cramps at the site of injection which last about 5 min, and are relieved by gentle massage and walking. The haemolysis induced by the hypertonic solution can lead to haemosiderin staining; this can be lessened by prior injection of air into the blood vessel. The other main problem with this sclerosant is the low but definite risk of superficial skin necrosis with sloughing and scarring if extravasation of the sclerosant occurs. Any extravasation of sclerosant should be immediately diluted with a large volume of normal saline or 1% lignocaine solution.

3 Aethoxysclerol (Polidocanol®) (Fig. 19.2) was initially developed as an anaesthetic agent, but it fell into disrepute when it was noted to have a sclerosant action on blood vessels. It is now used widely in Europe as the first choice of sclerosant, especially in Germany and France. Concentrations of 1–3% are used for the treatment of varicose veins, but it is better to use more dilute solutions (0.25–1.0%) when sclerosing small blood vessels. Aethoxysclerol has been reported as being almost free of toxicity with regard to pain and overlying necrosis. The incidence of allergic reactions also seems to be extremely low, although one non-fatal case of anaphylactic shock has been described following treatment for varicose veins. Post-sclerosis therapy pigmentation has been reported as frequently as 11%. The authors presently feel that it is the most suitable agent available, and should be used at a concentration of 0.25%, which reduces the incidence of slough and hyperpigmentation seen at higher concentrations.

Technique

It is important to inform the patient that the veins are likely to look much worse for a couple of weeks, and to explain that they should book the pro-

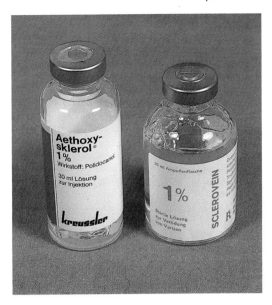

Fig. 19.2 Aethoxysclerol
preparations.

cedure 6–9 weeks away from any important social function. Injection of
sclerosant should be carried out with the patient in the supine position. The
skin is wiped with alcohol, which makes the skin more transparent, and
magnifiying glasses of 2–3 D also aid accurate cannulation of the vessels.
We advocate sclerosis of a small test area in a non-conspicuous site, before
going on to treat larger areas at each appointment. Cannulation of the vessels is easier with the needle bent to an angle of about 45° with the bevel
upwards, and if a small (2 ml) syringe is used (Fig. 19.3). The best needle is
probably a 32-gauge needle about 0.5 in long (Fig. 19.4). These needles
come with a fine stylet, to keep the needle patent, which should be
removed before use. Some surgeons prefer to inject a small bolus (up to
0.5 ml) of air into the blood vessel from the tip of the syringe after initial
cannulation of the vessel with the leg positioned so that the injection is
upwards, as blanching within the connected venous network indicates that
the vessel has been correctly cannulated. It also clears blood from the vessels, thus decreasing the risk of extravasation of red blood cells. It is clearly
best to pick out a reasonably large vessel at the centre of a group, which
serves as a feeder vessel for the group. For each group of vessels one can
inject between 0.1 and 0.5 ml; this should be enough to obliterate vessels
within a radius of up to 1 cm from the point of injection. After injection
with sclerosant the area becomes red and inflamed and takes on an urticarial response (Fig. 19.5) which may last several hours. The needle site should
be watched during injection so that injection can be stopped immediately
in case of extravasation. Muscle cramps usually resolve within 5 min.
If sclerosant does become extravasated, gentle massage, as opposed to rubbing, of the area for 60 s usually causes dispersion without serious problems. More serious extravasation of solution will result in acute pain
and burning, which may be relieved by aspirin or ice packs; dilution
of the sclerosant at the site is advised using physiological saline or 1%
lignocaine.

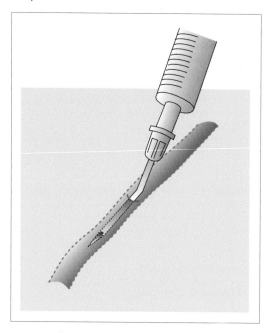

Fig. 19.3 Cannulation of vessel.

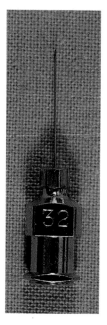

Fig. 19.4 Sclerotherapy
needle.

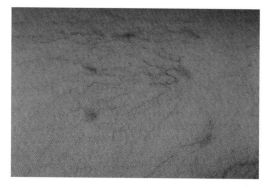

Fig. 19.5 Urticarial reaction
to sclerosant.

Patients should be told that there may be little obvious change in the vessels for up to 3 weeks, and that the procedure may need to be repeated several times. There is controversy as to whether patients should wear compression stockings for 72 h after sclerotherapy, such as Sigvaris® with a pressure of between 20 and 40 mmHg. Possible benefits would include keeping the irritated vessels sealed and reduction in thrombophlebitis and post-sclerosis hyperpigmentation. Treatments can be repeated every 3–4 weeks until the vessels have been adequately cleared.

Complications of sclerotherapy

The most common complication of sclerotherapy is that of hyperpigmentation along the course of the vessel; this tends to decrease over the first 6–9 months, but is sometimes permanent. Lower leg oedema can occur, especially after large volumes of sclerosant are used, deep vessel thrombophlebitis must be excluded. Thrombophlebitis is a rare problem; it is usually of the superficial type and often resolves spontaneously, but clearly the deep vein type will require anti-coagulation. Incision of a superficially thrombosed vessel with milking of the clot contents aids healing. Sloughing and scarring following extravasation occur to a greater extent with hypertonic saline. A fibrotic cord can occur after sclerosis of veins of 3–5 mm in diameter and can take more than 1 year to resolve. Acute allergic reactions and anaphylaxis can occur, and particular care needs to be exercised in those with a history of asthma.

A further complication is the development for unknown reasons of a network of small veins in the area 2–3 weeks following sclerotherapy. This is often seen by the patient as a recurrence of the original problem. Occasionally, these veins can be treated with further sclerotherapy.

19.4 Laser ablation

Telangiectatic vessels have in the past been treated, both on the face and on the lower legs, using the argon laser. There is, however, a risk of scarring and pigmentary change secondary to non-specific epidermal and upper dermal damage. Tunable pulsed dye lasers, where the laser-emitted energy is at a wavelength of 585 nm, produce selective vascular damage with hardly any scarring and have become the lasers of choice for treating vascular lesions including telangiectasia (see Chapter 20).

19.5 Improvement of actinic damage

The effects of sun exposure on the skin, including skin ageing, are now well established and are becoming well known by the public at large. Photoageing of the skin is characterised by wrinkling, increased laxity, yellowing, increased roughness, telangiectasia and spotty hyper- and hypopigmentation. The changes occur both in the epidermis and dermis, but much of the wrinkling and elastosis occurs from damage to elastic fibres in the dermis, which becomes thinner.

Photo-protection

Photo-protection is advisable for those who have skin types 1, 2 and 3 (Table 19.1) and consists of avoiding excessive solar exposure, especially

Table 19.1 Effects of sun exposure on skin type.

Skin type	Description
Type I	White skin; never tans, always burns
Type II	White skin; burns initially, tans with difficulty
Type III	White skin; tans easily, burns rarely
Type IV	White skin; never burns, always tans (Mediterranean type)
Type V	Brown skin; for example, Indian
Type VI	Black Afro-Caribbean skin

between 10:00 h and 16:00 h, the wearing of finely woven garments and broad-rimmed hats, and use of sunscreens of factor 15 and above.

Patients can sometimes be convinced of how much damage sun exposure is having on their skin by comparing sun-protected areas such as the medial upper arm with the skin on their face or dorsum of hands. Photo-protection guards not only against photo-ageing but also prevents actinic keratoses and basal and squamous cell epitheliomas.

Topical tretinoin

There is now increasing and convincing evidence that the use of topical tretinoin cream at a concentration of 0.1% significantly reduces many of the actinic changes described above. When used for some 16 weeks, photo-aged skin has been reported to show a definite reduction in fine wrinkles, a 70% decrease in discrete lentigines, and increased pinkness which enhances the appearance and makes the skin look more youthful. Cream can be applied daily for 3–6 months until adequate reversal of actinic damage has been shown, and then reduced to 0.05% cream for maintenance of the effects. Some patients do complain of dryness, erythema and flaking of the skin, burning, tingling or pruritus. These symptoms can be overcome by decreasing the frequency of application of the tretinoin, the use of emol-lients and very occasionally the use of a topical steroid preparation for a few days.

Skin peels

One of the most consistent and predictable ways of improving actinic dam-age in skin is to perform skin peeling. Skin peeling results in an increase in thickness of the papillary dermis, with the loss of some elastosis, and regen-eration of a normal epidermis. Removal of freckling, lentigines as well as seborrhoeic and actinic keratoses, also results in an improved skin appear-ance, and can reduce the number of times a patient requires treatment with liquid nitrogen or curettage and cautery for solar keratoses. The amount of change brought about depends on the depth of the chemical peel induced and the chemical agent used.

Alpha-hydroxyacids

The most superficial skin peels, amounting to a mild epidermolysis, can be achieved using alpha-hydroxyacids, which are a mixture of acids found in sugar cane as well as sour milk. Glycolic acid preparations are commercially available in concentrations of 20–70% (Neo Strata®, Gly Derm®) and peels with these agents may be carried out weekly at increasing concentra-tion. They have been used in the treatment of melasma, mild acne, wrin-kles and solar-induced pigmentary changes, and in conjunction with 5-fluorouracil in the treatment of actinic keratoses. Scarring has been recorded when the solutions have not been washed off after the recom-mended 3 min.

Superficial skin peels

Superficial peels carried out using concentrations of trichloroacetic acid between 20 and 35% can be used to treat light wrinkling and pigmentary changes due to actinic damage or cigarette smoking. There is evidence that the use of 0.05% tretinoin cream (Retinova®) for several weeks before a chemical peel increases the efficacy of the peel; used afterwards it can help to maintain the cosmetic improvement achieved from a peel. For deeper peels, either 50% trichloroacetic acid, or Baker's peel using phenol, can be carried out, but phenol peels can result in persistent hypertrophic scarring, irregular thinning and pigmentary changes, and should also be carried out only under cardiac monitoring. We will restrict further discussion to light to moderate chemical peeling with trichloroacetic acid. Trichloroacetic acid acts by precipitating epidermal proteins, thus causing necrosis and sloughing both of the normal and actinically damaged skin.

The skin on the area to be treated should first be degreased using topical alcohol or acetone. At this stage, use of Jessner's solution (Table 19.2) applied to the skin for a few minutes before the trichloroacetic acid results in a deeper peel. Alternatively, Jessner's solution may be used alone to induce a mild skin peel and has been used for the treatment of comedonal acne. For conditions such as melasma, two Jessner's peels may be applied, the second application being about 2 min after the first. For most chemical peels using trichloroacetic acid in concentrations less than 35%, analgesia is not required, but a nearby fan helps to keep the face cool and decrease patient discomfort. The stinging of the peel is directly proportional to the strength of trichloroacetic acid applied; treatments should be applied in segments which overlap slightly, so that no untreated areas occur. The peel agent is applied using a wrung-out damp gauze sponge or several cotton-tipped applicators at the same time, applying the agent as evenly as possible over the cosmetic unit to be peeled. With strong agents, frosting of the skin appears quickly (Fig. 19.6), but with weak agents this may not appear for 5 min. The peel should be carried through the hairline, the eyebrows and onto the vermilion border of the lips, so that an untreated line does not occur around these areas. The tragus and earlobe can also be peeled, and the peel can be tapered off below the jawline so that a cut-off line is not clearly observed. The eyelids should be peeled last, as they are most sensitive, and probably should not be peeled with greater than a 30% trichloroacetic acid solution. Peeling the eyelids should be carried out with a single cotton applicator or squirrel hairbrush, and can be taken up to 1 mm from the lid margin. The applicator used should be nearly dry so that it will not drip, and tears should be blotted by an assistant. If the agent does get into the eye, it is usually diluted to ineffectiveness, but clearly the eye should be flooded with water or saline.

Table 19.2 Jessner's solution.

Resorcinol	14 g
Salicylic acid	14 g
Lactic acid (85%)	14 g
Ethanol (95%)	Made up to 100 ml

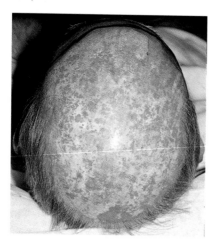

Fig. 19.6 Skin frosting following application of trichloroacetic acid peel to scalp.

Following the skin peel, the patient will complain of burning, heat or pain and some analgesia is usually required for 6–8 h. The following day, the face may be washed with water and an antibiotic ointment applied. Although complete healing may not be achieved for several months, the patient usually has an acceptable appearance and can wear light make-up after 1 month. Patients have increased sensitivity to sunlight and should stay out of the sun and use sunscreens following skin peeling.

Complications of chemical peels

One of the most feared complications of chemical peels is that of disseminated herpes simplex infection; patients must be treated prophylactically if there is a history of cold sores or herpetic lesions. With deeper chemical peels, hypopigmentation or hyperpigmentation can occur, and the risk of hyperpigmentation is increased with sun exposure. Lines of demarcation between peeled and unpeeled areas can lead to problems if the peel margin is not properly feathered. All patients will experience erythema, itching and burning in the first weeks, which can be helped by aspirin. Not uncommonly, however, this burning sensation and erythema lasts for several months, and is particularly noticeable when the patient is embarrassed or gets warm. In some cases, low-dose propranolol will help these symptoms.

Bacterial infections can occur, although they may be reduced in frequency by the use of a topical antibiotic. Infection with crusting can occur when the patient fails to follow instructions and has, on occasion, led to scarring.

Scarring following facial peels is infrequent, but the most common areas involved are on the upper lip and angle of jaw. Areas of slow healing or scabbing, detected early at the stage of 3 weeks postoperatively, may be treated with topical steroids which will often prevent scarring. For more established scars intralesional triamcinolone can be used.

Milia, prolonged erythema, pruritus, textural changes and skin atrophy are all recognised side effects.

Considerable time and effort should be devoted to informing patients about chemical peeling before the procedure is carried out; the patient should be fully informed of the pain and discomfort which will inevitably follow. Patients should be strongly motivated to have this form of therapy. However, if patients are willing to go through the associated postoperative discomfort, their facial appearance can be transformed and they will look younger.

Deep chemical peels

Deep chemical peels are induced using phenol or carbolic acids; the most common being the Baker's peel, which uses phenol in concentrations of around 50%. Patients require analgesia, intravenous fluids and, because of the risk of serious cardiac arrhythmias, cardiac monitoring during the procedure. The depth of the peel may be increased further by occlusion of the skin following application. These forms of peels can be associated with scarring and pigmentary disturbances and should only really be carried out by those with considerable experience of such procedures.

19.6 Filling agents

Indications for filling agents

Filling agents other than fat are usually used for the treatment of furrows, wrinkles and for augmentation of lips. The acne scars that are most responsive are those that are soft and have sloping borders; these are generally treated with Zyderm® 1 or 2 with 50–100% overcorrection to achieve the desired contour once fluid has been resorbed. For the treatment of wrinkles and soft scars, consideration must be given to the effects of gravity on the face. It is usually best to treat forehead creases with the patient supine and other areas on the face with the patient sitting near upright. Most patients can be injected without using any local anaesthetic, thus preventing distortion of the field. The only preparation required is that of washing the face to remove make-up and using alcohol wipes for antisepsis.

   A not uncommon problem with injecting material into the dermis is that when the needle lies within a sebaceous gland, the filling agent squirts out through the sebaceous ostium. When this happens, it is necessary to reposition the needle before further injection. Massage following injection can be used to even out the filling agent, rather than leaving a 'string of beads' effect. It is essential to slightly underfill a defect when using silicone as a filling agent and to treat at 4-weekly intervals until proper correction has been achieved, as silicone is a permanent implant. Another indication for the use of filling agents is after cosmetic or flap surgery, when irregularities in skin contours have developed.

Agents available

Collagen implants

The most commonly used filling agent in dermatological surgery is solubilised bovine dermal collagen, consisting of 95% type 1 collagen and

5% type 3 collagen. This is presently available as three separate products provided in prefilled syringes also containing lignocaine as a local anaesthetic.

The agents are as follows:

1 Zyderm® I with 35 mg/ml bovine dermal collagen;

2 Zyderm® II with 65 mg/ml bovine dermal collagen; and

3 Zyplast® which is a glutaraldehyde cross-linked collagen form that tends to shrink less and also last longer.

The use of each of these three products is to some extent determined by physician preference, but Zyderm® I tends to form tiny droplets when injected into the dermis giving a smoother overall result, whereas if Zyderm® II is placed high in the dermis it can sometimes be seen as creamy coloured plaques. Zyplast® is often seen as being lumpy when injected high in the dermis, although this settles with time. Zyderm® II and Zyplast® can be used to fill furrows, while Zyderm® I can be used to fill in finer skin creases. A slight overcorrection at the time of injection is required to take into account the resorption of the fluid excipient. If overcorrection is later found to be excessive, this can often be overcome by massage to reduce the size of the area. Following injection into the skin each of these forms of collagen gradually migrates deeper into the dermis and is finally extruded into the subcutaneous space, where it disappears over a period of 6–9 months. Persistence is longer over bony prominences and in and around scars, but the length of action of all of these forms of injectable collagen is limited to 3–9 months.

Skin testing

Allergy to this form of collagen is not insignificant; 10% of patients have collagen antibodies prior to its use and reactions occur in some 3–4% of patients. Because of this it is necessary to carry out a skin test using a small volume (0.1 ml) of the product injected into the inner forearm. Ninety per cent of those allergic to the product will react within 3–4 days and the rest will react within 4 weeks. The reactions are local, with inflammation and swelling, and only rarely leave scars. Because 2% of patients will react to treatment despite an initially negative skin test, many dermatologists carry out a second challenge 4 weeks later in the opposite arm or post-auricular area and wait for another 4 weeks before carrying out the treatment if there is again no reaction.

Injection technique

Local anaesthetic, if deemed necessary, may be injected around rather than into or under the scar or wrinkle to prevent distortions of the architecture. The needle is inserted a little way from the lesion and advanced at an angle of 45° under it, and the lesion is undermined by manipulating the needle in a 'fan-like' manner. The agent is then injected slowly until there is between 50 and 100% overcorrection of the defect, with elevation over the surrounding skin (Fig. 19.7b). Multiple punctures are best when using Zyderm® for fine wrinkles. For larger defects, the needle is advanced in the mid to deep dermis under the length of the lesion, while undermining with

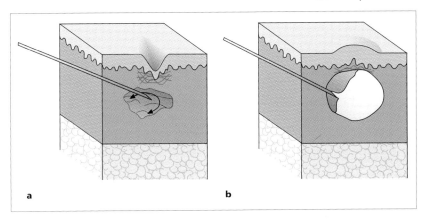

a   b

Fig. 19.7 (*Above*) Filling of skin depression. **a**. Creation of filling space by undermining. **b**. Overcorrection of defect.

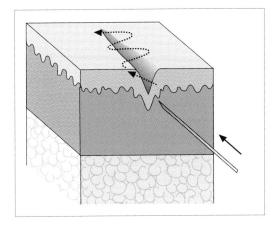

Fig. 19.8 Filling of linear depression by zigzag method.

a side to side motion; Zyderm® is then injected while withdrawing the needle. A modification of this technique involves advancing the needle in a zigzag manner from side to side across the defect, and withdrawing it in a similar fashion while injecting the Zyderm® (Fig. 19.8).

Injections need to be repeated after 2 weeks in up to 60% of patients. Corrections may last from 6 months to 1 year, but patients must appreciate that this is not a procedure which produces permanent results.

Complications of injected collagen

Local reactions. Patients must be informed of the fact that they can become allergic to collagen injections at any time during treatment. Allergy probably occurs in only 3% of patients undergoing soft tissue augmentation, and 90% of reactions occur with the first treatment. These reactions occur locally at the site of injection in the form of indurated, elevated, erythematous and pruritic areas. Nasolabial fold injections generally do not produce as much of a reaction as those at the glabella and forehead; at the glabella, fairly massive swelling, cyst formation and erythema may occasionally occur and lead to scarring. Most reactions fade gradually over 4–6 months, although some have lasted as long as 2 years. Some relief can be achieved with non-steroidal anti-inflammatory drugs

(NSAIDs); it is probably best not to give the patient systemic steroids as the doses required over long periods are not justified. More recently identified has been a vesicular and cystic reaction occurring more often with Zyplast® than with Zyderm®; cystic lesions should be drained to lessen the possibility of scarring.

Another side effect is that of intermittent swelling, observed in about 1% of treated patients, triggered by exercise, menstruation, alcohol or sun exposure. This reaction can last up to 3 years. It is felt that when the reaction has settled, patients can safely be treated again with Zyderm® without further problems.

Occasionally, where a lot of collagen has been injected into a small area, pressure necrosis will develop; this seems to be most common on the glabellar area. There has been one report of partial blindness following collagen injection in the glabellar area, probably as a result of retrograde embolisation by collagen solution.

Systemic reactions. Systemic reactions to injectable collagen have never been proven, although flu-like episodes have been reported in 0.1% of treatments. There is no substantive evidence that Zyderm® causes collagen vascular disease or dermatomyositis; the incidence of these conditions in patients receiving collagen injections is the same as in the general population. It is, however, clear that such agents should not be injected into a patient with a collagen vascular disease such as lupus erythematosus or scleroderma.

Silicone

The term silicone is used to describe a large family of polymers that contain silicon as their basic element. Dimethylpolysiloxsane (DMPS) polymer fulfils many of the criteria of an ideal implantable substance for soft tissue augmentation. It neither hardens nor softens with time, its viscosity remains constant, it is inert, tasteless and colourless and it does not elicit an immune reaction. In addition, it is relatively inexpensive, easily sterilised and stored, and when injected in small volumes is held in place by a strictly localised self-limited fibroblastic response without much of a foreign body or inflammatory response. The injectable form used is a highly purified DMPS which has been filtered to remove heavy metals and impurities, and has a viscosity of 350 cSt (centistoke; 3.5×10^{-4} m²/s).

Silicones have received bad press recently, stemming from the use of unpurified preparations, or the use of large volumes for soft tissue augmentation when movement of the silicone is a problem, and sudden death has been reported from intravascular embolisation. For this reason, both professional and public perception of silicone has been poor over recent years. Because of these concerns, in the USA silicones for injection currently do not have approval of the Food and Drug Administration. However, it seems likely that with the small volume injections used in dermatological surgery, the side effects are minimal. In the UK, the Committee on Safety of Medicines, after reviewing the available evidence, has not introduced any limitations on the use of silicone. Silicone seems safe if used in its absolutely pure form for small anatomical defects not involving glandular tissue. Because it is a permanent material which is not significantly resorbed, overcorrection of defects should not be undertaken; smaller 'microdroplet' injections with undercorrection should be used. The injections should be repeated at approximately 4-weekly intervals until the desired degree of correction has been achieved. Side effects include transient erythema, oedema, bruising and very occasionally intermittent swelling at the site of injection. Mild brown discoloration has been reported following the treatment of hypopigmented scars, and milder granulomatous reactions have been reported in 1:10 000 patients in association with a risk of infection or some form of allergic reaction.

Lipid injection

Lipid may be extracted by liposuction from one area of the patient's body, usually the abdomen or lateral thighs, and injected to correct defects, for example on the face. The donor area from which the fat is to be taken is injected with dilute lignocaine (0.25% or 0.5%) and anaesthesia is also achieved in the recipient area, using as little local anaesthetic as possible so as not to distort the anatomy. At the donor site a small incision is made. A 13–19-gauge blunt-ended needle, the syringe and a needle (Tulip® syringe and needle) fitted to a 10 or 20 ml syringe containing Ringer's lactate, is moved in and out of the fat with constant application of negative pressure on the syringe by aspiration; the donor skin is pinched between the fingers of the opposite hand so that as much fat as possible can be harvested, and about 4 ml should be taken into each syringe. When the syringe and needle are removed, the syringe is held with the needle down so that the fat floats to the top, while the redundant saline, blood and serous fluid can be disposed of, and the fat washed repeatedly with Ringer's lactate until clear. For implantation of fat a 16- or 18-gauge needle can be used. An overcorrection should be made to at least 100% when injecting, as over a few days swelling will resolve and the fat injected, which is an autologous transplant, will not all take. Once the fat has been injected it can be moulded by finger pressure and held in place with a dressing for a few days until fibrin clots stabilise the graft. While some corrections involving fat are long term, this is so in only about 50% of treated patients. Fat injections should not be used for wrinkles, but may be used to treat steroid atrophy, facial lipodystrophies and fat loss in the ageing face. Complications are few, and are restricted to bruising at the donor and recipient sites.

19.7 Dermabrasion

Dermabrasion is the abrasive technique used for the removal of superficial lesions, pitted or depressed scars, rhinophyma and tattoos. It is chiefly used on the face, where regeneration of the epidermis occurs quickly with minimal scarring. The area of skin to be treated with dermabrasion has to be frozen by a continuous stream of Freon® (dichlorotetrafluoroethylene), rendering the skin firm enough to be worked on. Dermabrasion is usually carried out with a hand-held dermabrader (Fig. 19.9a). Stainless steel wire

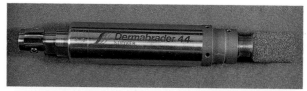

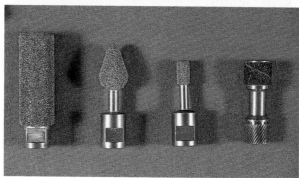

Fig. 19.9 Dermabrasion apparatus. **a.** Hand-held dermabrader. **b.** Selection of dermabrader heads.

brushes (Fig. 19.9b) or diamond fraizes are rotated by means of a high-speed rotary drill. Bleeding occurs for 15–30 min following treatment. After this, a topical antibiotic can be applied, over which a dressing of paraffin gauze or a non-adherent dressing is applied. Dressings should be removed in about 24 h, after which antibiotic ointment should be applied several times a day. Crusts separate from the area in around 7–10 days, with healing being complete within 3 weeks, particularly if the wound is left open and dry.

Surface refrigerants are frequently used as anaesthetics and they also provide the necessary skin firmness for dermabrasion. Some refrigerants have an excessive cooling effect, and their use may entail a risk of necrosis, scarring and loss of pigment.

In patients who are prone to cold sores, acyclovir prophylaxis is mandatory before and after treatment if a devastating herpes simplex infection is to be avoided. Mild irritation or discomfort from sunlight and cosmetics is likely to be present for a few months; patients must be warned to avoid these and to use a sunscreen with a high sun protection factor. Milia formation, persistent erythema, hyperpigmentation, hypertrophic scars and dermatitis are occasional complications. Black patients do well with dermabrasion, since although there is often very obvious hypopigmentation at around 6 weeks, there is often good return of pigmentation eventually. Asiatic skin is more difficult to control, and hypo- and hyperpigmentation can take some time to normalise. Dermabrasion should not be performed on a patient taking, or who has recently taken, isotretinoin, as this can lead to an increased incidence of keloid scarring.

Dermabrasion is carried out more frequently in the USA than in the UK; in the UK it is generally carried out by plastic surgeons under general anaesthetic. During the procedure there is widespread dissemination of blood, and this has led to practical problems in the prevention of hepatitis B and C infections and HIV infection in the surgeon and attendant staff. This requires the surgeon and staff to wear fully protective theatre suits complete with facial visor. Decontamination of the theatre is also required after the procedure. These considerations have seriously restricted the use of dermabrasion in many centres in recent years. Other disadvantages include the need for sophisticated equipment and skilled operating staff, the need for a skin refrigerant, which may produce pigmentary changes and the possibility of tearing skin in the peri-orbital and peri-oral regions.

A modification of the technique, known as manual dermabrasion, has recently been described. A dry wall/plaster sanding screen (medium grade, Fabricut®, 3 M), or silicone carbide sandpaper Tri-A-Mite®, 3 M is cut into rectangles measuring 2 × 3 in and steam autoclaved. This sanding paper is then wrapped around a 3-mm sterile syringe and after the area to be dermabraded has been anaesthetised with local anaesthetic, the area is gently abraded with a back and forth or circular motion until the skin is smoothed down to the level of the papillary dermis. This technique is particularly useful for improving scars following surgery, and can be performed some 6–12 weeks after the surgery. The advantages of manual dermabrasion are that it is less expensive, requires no specialist equipment or skin refrigerant and there are no aerosolised blood or tissue fragments which could infect theatre staff.

19.8 Liposuction

Liposuction is the removal of subcutaneous fat from the skin by means of a cannula attached to a suction device. Liposuction is most frequently carried out for cosmetic body contouring, for example in removing unwanted fat deposits on the abdomen, submental areas or thighs, or for the removal of more localised fat deposits such as lipomas, or in patients with gynaecomastia or lipodystrophies. In the preoperative assessment of the patient, it is important to exclude patients who have unrealistic expectations of liposuction, and patients should be warned that redistribution of fat to remaining fat cells can occur, especially with excessive calorie intake. Patients who must also be rigorously excluded are those with a bleeding diathesis, or currently on anti-coagulants, aspirin or NSAIDs. Patients taking oral contraceptives should stop the drug for 1 month before liposuction is undertaken.

Liposuction may be carried out either under general anaesthesia or following the injection of large volumes of low-concentration local anaesthetic (tumescent anaesthesia; see Chapter 5) and is usually now carried out by the 'dry technique', where only the negative suction pressure and mechanical rasping of fat with the cannula are used to remove fat cells. Local anaesthesia can be used on its own or with background general anaesthesia ('twilight sleep'); the use of a local anaesthetic in association with adrenaline solution decreases blood loss during the procedure, but the benefit of this may be outweighed by the increased length of the procedure.

The areas where fat is to be removed should be delineated with the patient standing, using a marker pen, and incision points for the cannula tip should also be marked and shown to the patient at the start of the procedure. After anaesthesia is induced, small incisions are made such as to allow the entrance of the cannula. Cannulae vary in length, diameter and size but should have blunt tips and apertures to the side. The cannula is attached to an aspiration pump usually operating at 1 atm of negative pressure. After insertion of the cannula through the entry point, it can be guided to the areas where fat is to be removed by the non-dominant hand, and fat is then systematically removed in a series of piston-like movements carried out in a criss-cross pattern; window-wiper-type sweeping movements should not be used.

During fat removal, the patient's blood pressure and pulse should be regularly monitored and for large volumes of fat removal the use of a pulse oximeter is recommended. Intravenous fluids may be necessary when more than 750 ml of fat is aspirated, especially in the elderly, and when volumes of fat exceeding 3 L are to be removed staged serial procedures are recommended.

Postoperatively, compression dressings should be applied to the areas that have undergone the fat removal to prevent bruising, haematoma or seroma formation, and extravasation of large amounts of fluid such as to cause hypovolaemia. Such compression can be applied either by using elastic taping or by specialised garments produced by a number of manufacturers. Some surgeons prescribe prophylactic antibiotics, usually cephalosporins, to prevent infection which may enter through the cannula ports. Postoperative complications can include bleeding, infection, surface dimpling or scar retraction. Discomfort and bruising frequently last for about 2 weeks, although residual tenderness may persist for months. Some patients will require further sculpturing procedures to achieve the desired surface contour. Limitations of the procedure include asymmetry, striae, skin ptosis and scarring at the points of cannula insertion.

Death following liposuction can occur as a consequence of overwhelming sepsis, hypovolaemia or fat embolism.

19.9 Cosmetic camouflage

Cosmetic camouflage is a useful technique to cover skin blemishes and conceal colour irregularities, which cannot otherwise be treated by surgical means. Camouflage can be used for the concealment of port wine stains, vitiligo, facial pigmentary abnormalities, tattoos and other lentigines. Cosmetic camouflage can also be used to good effect in concealing alopecia, for example by the proper pencilling of artificial eyebrows in patients with alopecia universalis.

Cosmetic camouflage can be especially helpful in disguising skin disfigurements in black skin. The psychological impact of pigmentary disturbance in black people can be profound; frequent causes include vitiligo, melasma, discoid lupus and other inflammatory disorders which may not be noticed in skin types 1 and 2. Because black skins are uniquely multi-hued, at least 35 shades of pigmentation ranging from cream to brown and ebony are required. Unfortunately, only a limited number of cosmetic companies have ventured into this market. However, suitable preparations are available from Dermablend®, Fashion Fair®, Lydia O'Leary® and Clinique®.

Cosmetic camouflage is best left to trained personnel who can advise on colour match and colour blending. Several products are presently on the market including Dermablend® (10 shades), Dermacolour® (55 shades)

Table 19.3 Colour opposites used in the masking of cosmetic blemishes.

Blemish colour	Masking colour
Blue	Orange
Red	Green
Yellow	Purple

and Keromask® (11 shades). These are now prescribable on the National Health Service tariff in the UK and advice regarding proper blending is often available through the voluntary services of the British Red Cross. For corrective camouflage cosmetics it is necessary to use a colour selection opposite to the primary colour of the blemish. The colour opposites are shown in Table 19.3. Thus, a post-peel patient with red skin may find that a lime green product is the best form of camouflage. It is important not to overapply the agent when applying camouflage, as this will lead to a theatrical or clown-like look; 80% coverage is all that is required for everyday activities. The camouflage should be applied using a make-up sponge; the skin is rolled and dabbed gently, and applications are repeated until the area is covered. Fingers and brushes are not satisfactory methods of application. Most of the masking covers are available in all skin tones, are waterproof and long lasting. Many require only minor touching-up every few days. They have a high degree of patient acceptance and usually result in improved emotional well-being and attitude to everyday life. Most are non-comedogenic and have a low incidence of sensitisation; they do vary in their oiliness. Some have sunscreens incorporated, which makes them more useful for some patients, for example those with vitiligo or who have post-chemical peel.

Bibliography

Allerton EP. Cosmetics in blacks. *Dermatol Clin* 1991; 9: 53–68.

American Academy of Dermatology Advisory Board and members of the CTFA Task Force on Cosmetics. A primer on cosmetics. *J Am Acad Dermatol* 1992; 27: 469–84.

Asken S. Refinements in the technique of liposuction. *J Dermatol Surg Oncol* 1988; 14: 1165–72.

Brody HJ. *Chemical Peeling*. St. Louis: Mosby Year Book, 1992.

Coleman WP. The dermatologist as a liposuction surgeon. *J Dermatol Surg Oncol* 1988; 14: 1057–8.

Dolsky RL, Asken S, Nguyen A. Surgical removal of lipomas by lipo-suction surgery. *Am J Cosmet Surg* 1986; 3: 27–34.

Drake LA, Ceilly RI, Cornelison RL *et al.* Guidelines of care for dermabrasion. *J Am Acad Dermatol* 1994; 31: 654–7.

Duffy DM. Silicone: a critical review. In: Callen JP., ed. *Advanced Dermatology*, Vol. 5. Chicago: Year Book Medical Publishers, 1990.

Dzubow LM. Survey of refrigeration and surgical techniques used for facial dermabrasion. *J Am Acad Dermatol* 1985; 13: 287–92.

Ellis CN, Weiss JS, Hamilton TA, Headington JT, Zelickson AS, Voorhees JJ. Sustained improvement with prolonged topical tretinoin (retinoic acid) for photoaged skin. *J Am Acad Dermatol* 1990; 23: 629–37.

Elson ML. Correction of dermal contour defects with the injectable collagens: choosing and using these materials. *Semin Dermatol* 1987; 6: 77–82.

Elson ML. Collagen implantation. In: Harahap M, ed. *Complications of Dermatological Surgery*. Berlin: Springer-Verlag, 1993.

Engasser PG. Cosmetics and contact dermatitis. *Dermatol Clin* 1991; 9: 67–77.

Field LM. Liposuction surgery (suction-assisted lipectomy). *Semin Dermatol* 1987; 6: 214–27.

Fournier PF. Who should do syringe liposculpturing? *J Dermatol Surg Oncol* 1988; 14: 1055–6.

Goldman MP, Bennett RG. Treatment of telangiectasia. *J Am Acad Dermatol* 1987; 17: 167–82.

Goldman MP, Martin DE, Fitzpatrick RE, Ruiz-Esparza J. Pulse dye laser treatment of telangiectases with and without subtherapeutic sclerotherapy. *J Am Acad Dermatol* 1990; 23: 23–30.

Gonzalez E, Gange RW, Momtaz KT. Treatment of telangiectases and other benign vascular lesions with the 577 nm pulsed dye laser. *J Am Acad Dermatol* 1992; 27: 220–6.

Hanke CW, Roenigk H Jr, Pinski JB. Complications of dermabrasion resulting from excessively cold skin refrigeration. *J Dermatol Surg Oncol* 1985; 11: 896–900.

Kadunce DP, Burr R, Gress R, Kanner R, Lyon JL, Zone JJ. Cigarette smoking: risk factor for premature facial wrinkling. *Ann Intern Med* 1991; 114: 840–4.

Lillis PJ. Liposuction surgery under local anaesthetic: limited blood loss and minimal lidocaine absorption. *J Dermatol Surg Oncol* 1988; 14: 1145–8.

Ross RM, Johnson GW. Fat embolism after liposuction. *Chest* 1988; 93: 1294–5.

Rubenstein R, Roenigk HH, Stegman SJ *et al*. Atypical keloid after dermabrasion of a patient taking isotretinoin. *J Am Acad Dermatol* 1986; 15: 280–5.

Rubin MG. *Manual of Chemical Peels. Superficial and Medium Depth*. Philadelphia: JB Lippincott, 1995.

Stegman SJ, Tromovitch TA, Glogau RG. *Cosmetic Dermatological Surgery*. Chicago: Year Book Medical Publishers, 1990.

Weinstein GD, Nigra TP, Pochi PE *et al*. Topical tretinoin for treatment of photodamaged skin: a multicenter study. *Arch Dermatol* 1991; 127: 659–65.

Weiss JS, Ellis CN, Headington JT, Tincoff T, Hamilton JA, Voorhees JJ. Topical tretinoin improves photoaged skin. *J Am Med Assoc* 1988; 259: 527–32.

Zisser M, Kaplan B, Moy RL. Surgical pearl: manual dermabrasion. *J Am Acad Dermatol* 1995; 33: 105–6.

20 Advanced techniques

20.1 Closure of sides of unequal length

Many fusiform wounds or flaps involve the suturing together of wound margins that are not of the same length. When the lengths of the opposing sides of the wound are not greatly different, it is often possible to close the wound without redesigning its configuration by using the technique of halving.

Technique of halving

In this simple technique, skin on the longer side of the wound is distributed evenly over the entire length of the shorter side of the wound. The first suture is placed in the centre of each excisional margin, while the second and subsequent sutures continue to divide the residual defects into equal smaller compartments in a similar manner (Fig. 20.1). Because of the elasticity of the skin, the shorter side tends to stretch to match that of the longer, without noticeable puckering in the wound.

Where the edges of the wound are more disproportionate, a 'dog-ear' or Von Burow's triangle repair may be required.

'Dog-ear' repairs

Where the angle at the apices of an ellipse excision is greater than 30°, there will be a tendency for bunching up of excess tissue at either end of the wound closure, resulting in a 'dog-ear' (Fig. 20.2). It is sometimes possible to control the 'dog-ear' simply by placing sutures over it, especially in the elderly where the skin is quite forgiving. For larger 'dog-ears', or those occurring in younger patients, repair can be carried out in a number of ways, all of which yield a good cosmetic result. The choice of technique will depend on the exact situation.

Perhaps the simplest technique is to use a skin hook placed in the apex of the 'dog-ear' to pull the redundant tissue to one side such that its base lies in the line of the wound (Fig. 20.3). The exposed side of the base of the 'dog-ear' is then cut with a scalpel along the line of the wound, and the partially transected redundant piece of tissue is pulled to the opposite side of the wound. A second incision is made along the base of the 'dog-ear' as before, to the apex of the first incision (Fig. 20.4), and the triangular piece of redundant tissue is then discarded. The wound may now be sutured in the normal way.

'Dog-ears' can also be removed by creating two small triangles by dividing the apex of the 'dog-ear' in half with a scalpel. The redundant tissue from each side is then in turn pulled over the line of the wound and removed after incising its base before standard wound closure. 'Dog-ears'

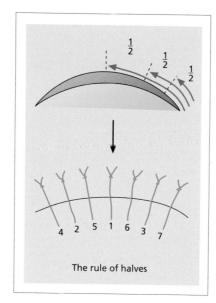

The rule of halves

Fig. 20.1 Wound closure by rule of halves.

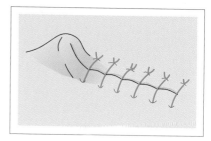

Fig. 20.2 'Dog-ear' at end of wound.

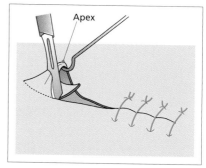

Fig. 20.3 Excess skin of 'dog-ear' pulled to one side using skin hook and incised to apex in line with the original incision.

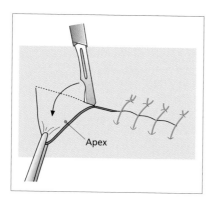

Fig. 20.4 The redundant skin pulled to the opposite side of the wound using tissue forceps and incised to the apex along the direction of the initial incision.

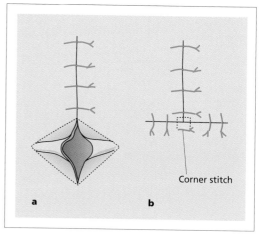

Fig. 20.5 Excision of 'dog-ear' by T-plasty.

may also be removed by excising the redundant tissue as a new ellipse, thus extending the original incision line but keeping it in the same direction. Alternatively, the 'dog-ear' can be converted into a 'T' and the excess skin removed as in a T-plasty (Fig. 20.5) The junction of the long and short arms of the 'T' should be sutured using a four-point suture. Other variations on 'dog-ear' repair include curved (Fig. 20.6), L-shaped (Fig. 20.7) and V-shaped (Fig. 20.8) repairs. The latter is a useful technique when the length of the wound cannot be extended.

Von Burow's triangle

Another method of closing a wound with sides of unequal length is to excise a small triangular piece of tissue (Von Burow's triangle) from the longer side, thereby decreasing its length (Fig. 20.9). This excision is usually done at either end of the wound, but can be carried out anywhere along the length of the longer side, such that the linear closure that results from

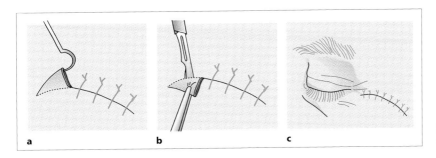

Fig. 20.6 Curved 'dog-ear' repair.

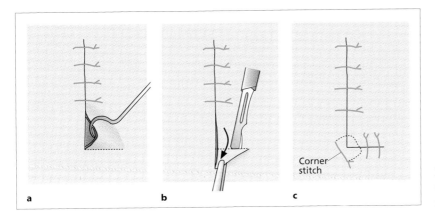

Fig. 20.7 L-shaped 'dog-ear' repair.

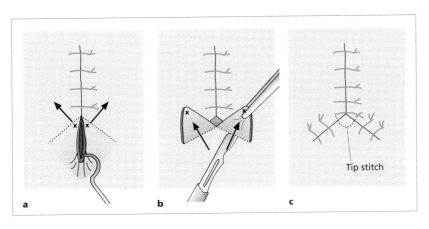

Fig. 20.8 V-shaped 'dog-ear' repair.

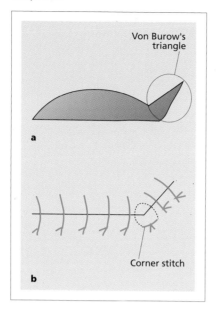

Fig. 20.9 Closure of wound with sides of unequal length by using Von Burow's triangle.

the triangular excision can be hidden in an appropriate anatomical line or fold. The junction of the main wound margins with those of the excised triangle should again be secured with a four-point suture.

20.2 Partial and combined wound closure

In certain circumstances, for example due to excessive tension in a wound, it may not be desirable to completely close the wound by suturing. In such situations, it may be possible to use a combination of methods of wound closure, such as suturing part of the wound and allowing the remainder to heal by secondary intention.

Close to cosmetically important borders, for example around the lips, healing by secondary intention could result in contractures and undesirable functional and aesthetic effects. The margins of the wound may be approximated at the ends, leaving the centre to heal by secondary intention. 'Guiding sutures' may be placed across the area of a wound which is being left to heal by secondary intention, which has the effect of directing tension away from cosmetically or functionally important borders, thus preventing distortion during the phase of wound contraction.

A variation of the partial closure of a wound is the combined closure technique, in which excess skin, usually in the form of 'dog-ears', is removed, defatted and sown into place as a full thickness graft at the centre of the wound, where tension is greatest. This has the advantage of providing wound closure using a skin graft of matching skin, without the need to harvest a skin graft from another site.

20.3 M-Plasty

It is sometimes not possible to complete an ellipse excision of a lesion without crossing an important anatomical or cosmetic line. The use of an M-

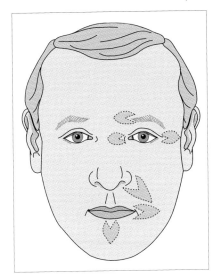

Fig. 20.10 Sites where M-plasty is suitable.

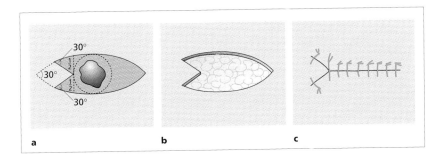

Fig. 20.11 Technique of M-plasty.

plasty conserves tissue and reduces the length of the excision line. This type of repair is particularly useful around the anatomical borders at the medial and lateral canthi of the eye, the eyebrows, around the lips and at the side of the nose (Fig. 20.10). The M-plasty repair may be performed at one or both ends of the excision. When planning to excise a malignant lesion using an M-plasty it is important to make sure that the point of the M does not compromise the planned excision margin. To perform an M-plasty repair it is best to draw a standard ellipse on the skin lesion with the apices being at angles of 30° (Fig. 20.11). At the apex where the M-plasty is required, two lines, each at 30° angles and inset into the apex of the ellipse, are drawn to complete the 'M'. Excision is then carried out. When suturing the resultant defect with a three-point corner suture to the M-plasty tip, it is wise to counteract the inevitable retractions by inserting the needle into either side of the main wound margin slightly ahead of its location in the M-plasty tip.

20.4 Z-Plasty

The Z-plasty is a technique which has become established in the treatment of contractures and in the management of facial scars, and enables the

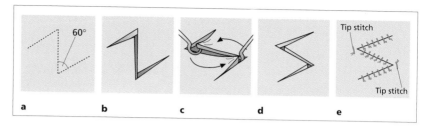

Fig. 20.12 Technique of Z-plasty.

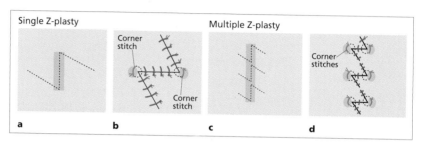

Fig. 20.13 Technique of Z-plasty. **a, b**. Single Z-plasty. **c, d**. Multiple Z-plasty. Note breaking up of zone of lateral tension (shaded areas) with multiple Z-plasty.

surgeon to break up and change the direction of a scar to give the best cosmetic result (Fig. 20.12). The angle size used in the Z-plasty will determine the percentage lengthening that can be expected; with an angle of 30° there is a theoretical 25% increase in the length of a wound, with 45° a 50% increase and with 60° a 75% increase. The standard angle size used for a Z-plasty is 60°; lesser angles do not produce a worthwhile increase in length, and may lead to poor blood supply to the flap, while greater angles lead to excessive transverse shortening. While the angle size controls the percentage increase in the length of a limb of the Z-plasty, the actual length of the wound increases proportionately with increase in the original limb length.

Use of multiple Z-plasty to break up a facial scar, or suture a wound which is under some tension, enables reduction in the amount of transverse shortening without significantly affecting the amount of lengthening. The net effect is to break up a long scar, with tension directly along the wound, into multiple short scars in which the tension has been redistributed such that the greater part of the shearing strain is taken up by the transverse limbs of the Z-plasties (Fig. 20.13).

20.5 Meshed wound closure

Where the tension in the centre of an ellipse is such as to prevent primary wound closure by using a simple line of sutures, for example with a wide ellipse excision of a lesion on the lower leg, the meshed wound closure technique can be employed. A number of short (1 cm) tension-relieving incisions in the surrounding skin, 1 cm apart and 1 cm from the wound margin, are made parallel to the sides of the intended wound closure. The

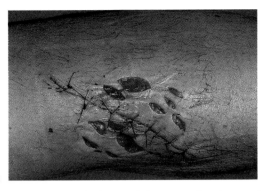
a

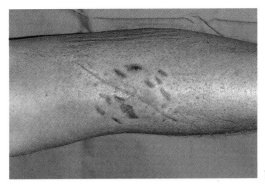
b

Fig. 20.14 Meshed wound closure: **a**. showing tension-relieving incisions to enable the wound to be closed centrally and **b**. healing at 2 weeks.

wound margins are partially approximated following extensive undermining, and are sutured freely and without tension, without necessarily closing the primary defect. The linear tension-relieving incisions open up as secondary ellipses, which are then allowed to heal by secondary intention (Fig. 20.14). The whole area is dressed with an antibiotic ointment or iodine-impregnated dressing changed once or twice weekly until the secondary ellipses have healed, usually over 4–6 weeks' time. This method of wound closure is preferable to closing an ellipse on the lower leg under tension, which might lead to tissue anoxia, necrosis and breaking down of the wound. The appearances are usually better than after skin grafting or healing by secondary intention, although the patient should be warned that multiple small scars will result.

20.6 Wedge resection of ear

Wedge resections of the external ear are particularly useful for large basal or squamous cell carcinomas affecting the pinna. A wedge resection of the ear allows the removal of such lesions under local anaesthesia by performing a ring block of the ear as described in Chapter 5. The external auditory canal should be packed with sterile cotton wool or a dental roll before starting surgery, to prevent it filling with blood during the procedure. For slender wedges of the ear which are extended down to the concha it is often possible to approximate the edges of the wound without causing buckling, deformity and lateral protrusion of the helix (Fig. 20.15a). Where such deformity does occur, this can be corrected by the use of stellate tension-relaxing excisions (Fig. 20.15b). Such stellate excisions are created by the placement of V-shaped wedges with a long axis perpendicular to the margins of the primary excision, and are placed near the mid-portions of the original wedge, usually in the anti-helix. It is best to make the secondary wedges smaller initially, since they can be extended at a later stage, if necessary, to achieve optimum closure of the wound. An example of a V-shaped wedge excision is shown in Fig. 20.16. Skin hooks can be used to approximate the margins of the helix until it is decided that no further modifications of the secondary wedges are required. Haemostasis can be

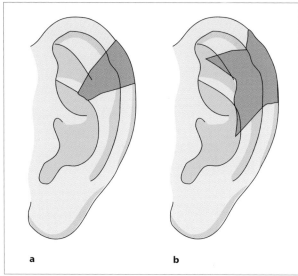

Fig. 20.15 Design of wedge excision of ear. **a**. V-shaped excision and **b**. Stellate tension-relaxing excision.

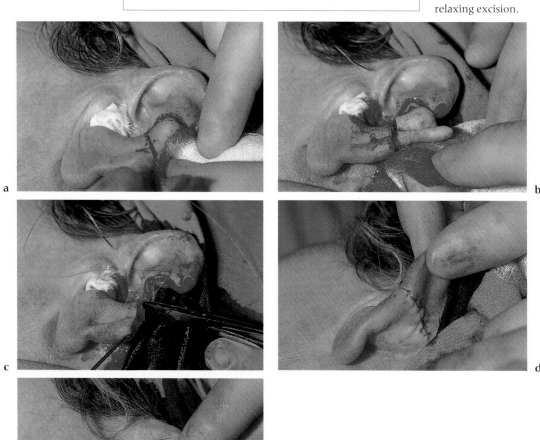

Fig. 20.16 Wedge resection of ear for chondrodermatitis nodularis helicis. **a**. V-shaped wedge cut from ear. (Note cotton wool plug in external auditory meatus.) **b**. Removal of wedge. **c**. Suture of cartilage with absorbable sutures. **d**, **e**. Suturing of posterior and anterior aspects of ear.

achieved using electrosurgery, but care should be taken to minimise damage to cartilage which might result in necrosis. Subcutaneous absorbable sutures such as 5/0 Vicryl® can be used to approximate the auricular cartilage. If undermining of the skin is required along the margins to achieve skin closure, care should be taken to remain above the perichondrium. The skin can then be closed, if necessary, using interrupted vertical mattress 6/0 synthetic sutures to achieve eversion of the wound.

As a dressing, the wound can be covered with antibiotic ointment and a non-adherent gauze. The concha is filled with a cotton wool ball, and gauze is placed in the post-auricular region, with a mild pressure bandage being applied around the head. The latter can be removed after 24–48 h. The sutures may be removed in 7–10 days.

20.7 Wedge resection of lip

A wedge resection of the lip is often required for the treatment of an invasive squamous cell carcinoma of the lower lip. Up to one-third of the lower lip can be resected as a 'V', and the defect closed directly, without functionally constricting the oral aperture. This method is particularly useful for squamous cell carcinomas in the centre of the lower lip, and is illustrated in Fig. 20.17.

Anaesthesia can be achieved either by bilateral mental blocks (see Chapter 5) or by local infiltration with anaesthetic. The anterior buccal sulcus can be packed with sterile gauze, or suction apparatus used, to control blood entering the mouth during the procedure. To limit bleeding, before the skin incisions are made, large synthetic sutures may be inserted through the lip, lateral to the wedge to be removed on each side, to a depth such as to close off the inferior labial artery. This helps the surgeon to clip and subsequently tie these vessels, rather than having to control them after they have been transected. The junction between the vermilion and the skin of the lip should be marked on either side, just lateral to the proposed excision, with sutures, to enable correct reapproximation (Fig. 20.17b). It may be helpful to design an M-plasty or Z-plasty at the lower part of the excision to prevent extension of the scar beyond the mental crease.

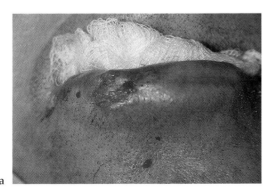
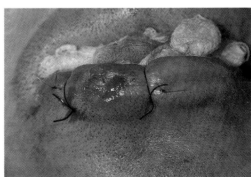

a   b

Fig. 20.17 Wedge excision of lip for squamous cell carcinoma. **a**. Original lesion. **b**. Gauze packing of the anterior buccal sulcus, with lateral sutures marking vermillion border and large diameter sutures to limit bleeding.

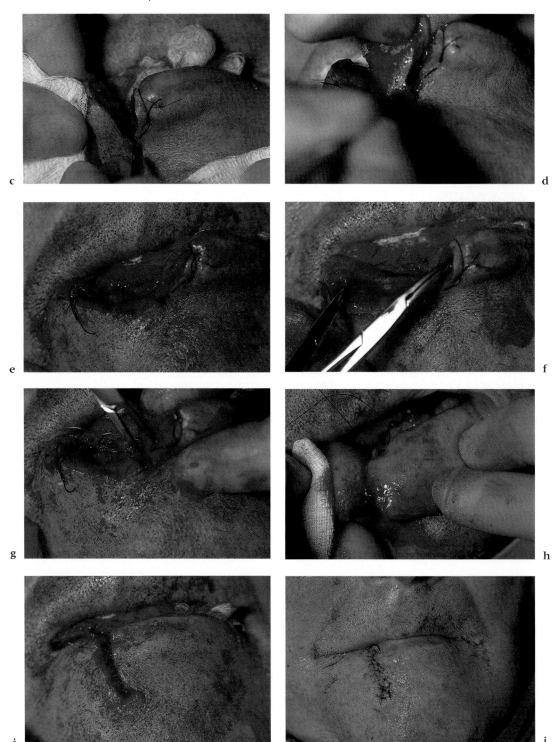

Fig. 20.17 *Continued* **c**. Initial incision; **d**. wedge incision completed; **e**. resultant defect; **f**. artery forceps applied to severed inferior labial artery; **g**. suturing of the muscle layer using absorbable sutures; **h**. suturing of labial mucous membrane using silk sutures; and **i**, **j**. suturing of skin wound.

The wedge of lip is most easily excised by having an assistant hold one lip edge under tension while the surgeon holds the other edge under tension. The length of the incision on the mucous membrane should not usually be as great as that on the skin surface. The severed ends of the inferior labial artery must be quickly clamped before they retract, and tied off with 4/0 Vicryl® sutures (Fig. 20.17f). Electrocautery can then be used on smaller vessels. It is important that the resultant defect is closed in layers. The deep muscle fascia is first sutured using interrupted buried 5/0 Vicryl® sutures. The labial mucous membrane is then sutured in a similar manner with silk sutures (Fig. 20.17h). The vermilion border is now closed with 5/0 silk interrupted sutures (for patient comfort), or perhaps more practically, 6/0 monofilament nylon sutures, with careful reapproximation of the vermilion–cutaneous border. Finally, the skin is closed with monofilament nylon sutures (Fig. 20.17i,j).

20.8 Mucosal advancement of lip

Removal of the vermilion area of the lower lip with advancement of the adjacent buccal mucous membrane to cover the defect can be a very effective method of treating extensive active cheilitis or early squamous cell carcinoma. Patients should be warned to use lip gloss incorporating a potent sunscreen, post surgery. The procedure is illustrated in Fig. 20.18.

The area to be excised includes that between the vermilion–cutaneous border and the line along which the upper and lower lips oppose when the mouth is closed.

Following removal of the vermilion down to the submucosa (Fig. 20.18b), the buccal mucous membrane may be undermined in the same plane above the orbicularis oris muscle as far as necessary, to provide a flap of mucosa adequate to cover the defect without undue tension. The flap is pulled forwards, with the aid of skin hooks, if necessary, and anchored in place with subcutaneous absorbable sutures (Fig. 20.18c,d) to approximate with the line of the previous vermilion–cutaneous border. Precise refashioning of the border is carried out by the rule of halving, using interrupted silk sutures.

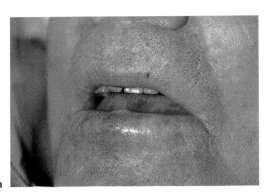
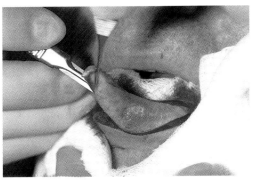

a   b

Fig. 20.18 Mucosal advancement of lip for squamous cell carcinoma. **a**. Initial lesion. **b**. Excision of lip mucosa along the vermilion border.

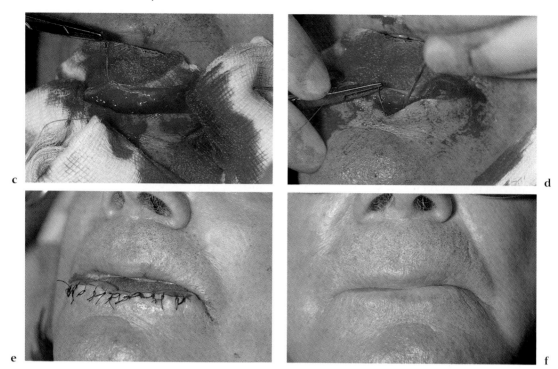

Fig. 20.18 *Continued* **c, d**. Approximation of new mucosal surface to skin with subcutaneous absorbable sutures. **e**. Silk sutures to close defect. **f**. Final result at 3 months.

20.9 Skin grafts

Skin grafts are of two kinds.

1 Whole skin grafts (Wolfe graft, pinch grafts) consisting of epidermis and full thickness dermis.

2 Split skin grafts consisting of epidermis and a variable amount of dermis as usually cut using a dermatome.

Whole skin grafts are suitable for small defects, since the graft remains virtually at its original size, whereas split skin grafts are more suited to wounds requiring large areas of skin cover and are subject to wound contraction.

The graft adheres to its bed initially by fibrin adhesion, with the nutritional requirements being met by diffusion from the graft bed. Outgrowth of capillary buds from the recipient graft bed into the graft occurs as early as 3 days, after which the strength of the attachment increases quickly, although it takes much longer for lymphatic drainage and nerve supply to be re-established.

For a graft to take, the graft bed must be capable of producing granulation tissue readily, and must be free of infection. Muscle and fascia generally accept grafts readily, as does fat on the face, which is extremely vascular; fat on other sites has a relatively poor vascular supply, leading to poor graft take. Cartilage covered with perichondrium, bone covered by periosteum and tendon covered with paratendon all accept grafts readily.

Full thickness grafts (Wolfe graft)

Wolfe grafts are commonly used to cover wounds that cannot be closed by primary suture or by using a flap, or which occur in areas such as the tip of the nose or the lower eyelid, where wound contracture could give rise to deformity of an important anatomical border. Whole skin grafts for the face are often taken from the post-auricular skin, which has the advantage of being hairless and which provides good skin colour and texture match when replacing facial skin. Other areas where skin can be harvested for replacement of facial skin include the upper eyelid and the supraclavicular fossa, although the latter tends not to give as good a colour or texture match as post-auricular skin. Examples of full thickness grafts are shown in Figs 20.19 and 20.20. The size of the graft required can be determined by making a template of the wound to be covered; such a template can be easily made from the sterile cardboard taken from a suture pack (see Fig. 20.19b,c). The graft skin is then excised to the level of the fat from the donor area. It is important to completely defat the underside of the graft with scissors once it has been removed (see Fig. 20.19e). The graft is then sown circumferentially into place using interrupted sutures (see Fig. 20.19f,g). The cut end of the sutures should be kept long, so that they can be tied over a small tissue buttress, usually made from sterile cotton wool, which is placed on the graft following the initial application of paraffin gauze layers (see Fig. 20.19h). The buttress has the effect of allowing the graft to be held firmly against the graft bed, and also to immobilise it, and thus reduces shearing strains which might otherwise lead to graft sliding on

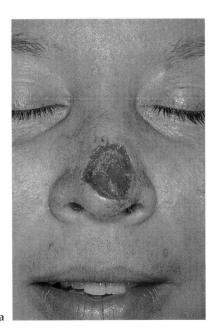
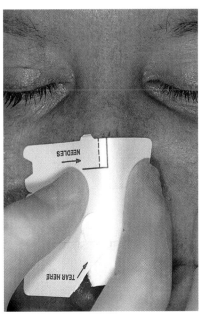

a   b

Fig. 20.19 Full thickness (Wolfe) graft to nose. **a.** Original defect; **b, c.** fashioning of template.

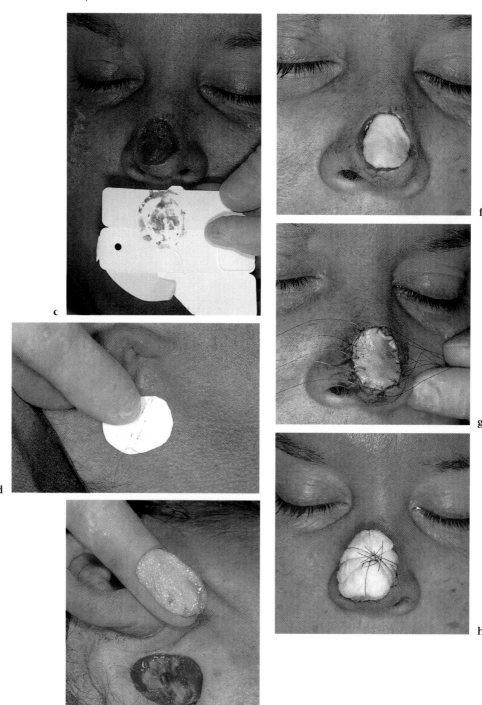

Fig. 20.19 *Continued* **d**. application of template to post-auricular skin; **e**. defatted graft after removal from donor site; **f**. placement of graft on defect; **g**. suture of grafting into place; and **h**. sutures tied centrally to hold buttress in place.

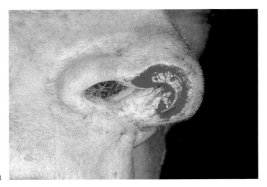
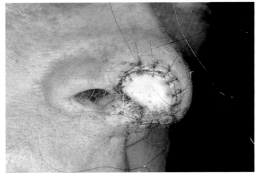
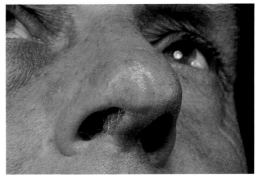

Fig. 20.20 Full thickness graft to nose. **a**. Original defect; **b**. graft sutured in place; and **c**. cosmetic appearance at 3 months.

the bed before there is strong fibrous tissue anchorage. The sutures may alternatively be secured in place above the buttress using a bead-and-collar tie-over. The long suture ends are pulled through the bead-and-collar and the bead is then fixed in position by crushing the metal collar with a needle holder.

The donor area for full thickness skin grafts is then closed using conventional closure techniques.

Pinch grafts

The technique of pinch grafting has been used most successfully in the treatment of leg ulcers, where the final cosmetic appearance is usually not so important, and where other forms of grafts usually fail due to the exudate formed from the wound. For pinch grafts to take, it is essential that the wound is first swabbed to make sure that there is no infection present; if there is, it should be treated, if necessary, with systemic antibiotics until three negative swabs are achieved. Pinch grafts are usually taken from the anterior thigh. A large rectangular area is anaesthetised by a field block using 0.5% lignocaine with adrenaline. Small pinch grafts (5–10 mm) can then be harvested by picking up small amounts of skin with a needle and shaving the tented skin off with a scalpel. The grafts are then placed on the granulating ulcer bed in close approximation with one another. The resulting cobblestone-like grafts are held in place under a paraffin gauze dressing, which is in turn immobilised under a layer of gamgee and a firm support dressing from forefoot to below knee. This dressing is left on for around 10

227

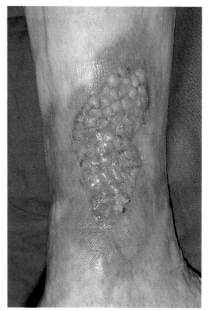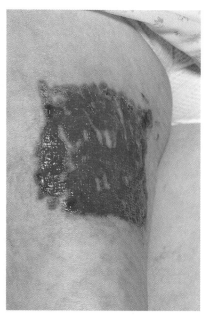

a

b

Fig. 20.21 a. Pinch grafts on venous leg ulcer after 10 days. **b**. Donor site healing by granulation at 10 days.

days (Fig. 20.21). The donor site can initially be dressed with Kaltostat® under a non-adherent dressing, held in place with a firm support dressing for a few days to achieve haemostasis. This can then be soaked off, and the area allowed to heal by granulation (Fig. 20.21b) under a paraffin gauze dressing.

Split skin grafts

Split skin grafts are usually used to cover large wounds, and are usually taken using a dermatome, which has a gauge allowing the surgeon to determine the thickness of the graft. The split skin graft can be applied to a raw surgically created surface or to a clean granulating wound. This type of skin grafting is very useful, and while not usually undertaken by dermatological surgeons, is a technique with which they should be familiar and should consider using when necessary.

20.10 Cutaneous random pattern skin flaps

Increasingly, dermatological surgeons are using local random pattern flaps for the closure of wound defects. Such flaps depend for their perfusion on the rich vascular network of the subdermal plexus, especially on the face and scalp. This random nature of the vascular pattern does place limitations on the dimensions, particularly the length:breadth ratio, of such flaps. Occasionally, axial pattern flaps can be designed where a recognised arteriovenous system runs along the length of the flap, allowing it to be of greater length than a random pattern flap. An example of this is a nasolabial flap based on the terminal branches of the angular artery.

General considerations in flap surgery

There are many types of flap described, with almost infinite variations. Described are some flaps to illustrate the general principles of flap surgery. The advantage of flap surgery is that the aesthetic appearance is usually better than that associated with a free graft, as there will usually be a much better skin match to the surrounding tissue. The disadvantage is that if a flap is not properly planned, then ischaemia, haematoma formation or infection may give rise to flap failure. This may require replacement of the flap with a skin graft, or more usually the removal of necrotic tissue by debridement, allowing the area to heal by secondary intention. Flap failure is more common in patients who smoke, who are diabetic, have a bleeding diathesis or are on anti-coagulant therapy.

Advancement flaps

Advancement flaps are probably among the most common type of flap used by dermatological surgeons. Advancement flaps characteristically move in a straight line, with the flap tissue stretching over the defect, and the wound being closed by one of the methods of unequal side closure (see above). Undermining should be carried out at the level of the subcutaneous fat.

Single advancement flap

The single advancement flap is one of the simplest flaps to use, and enables incision lines to be orientated to fit into natural folds. Generally, this form of flap should have a length:width ratio of no more than 3:1 in order to maintain sufficient vascular supply and avoid compromising the viability of the tip of the flap (Fig. 20.22). It may be necessary to remove a Von Burow's triangle on either side of the pedicle. This flap can be used on the upper bridge of the nose, or occasionally on the eyebrows.

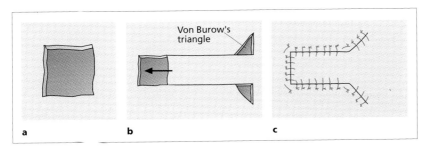

Fig. 20.22 Single advancement flap. **a.** Defect; **b.** creation of flap for advancement; and **c.** suturing of flap in place.

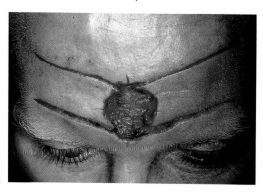

a

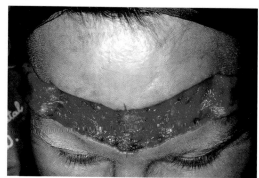

b

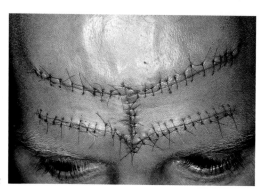

c

Fig. 20.23 Double advancement flap. **a**. Central defect following Mohs' surgery with incisions for bilateral advancement flaps; **b**. mobilisation of flaps by undermining; and **c**. flaps sutured in place.

Double advancement flap

The double advancement flap (Fig. 20.23) is commonly used to close defects on the forehead where the incisions can be located in the transverse creases, or for the upper eyebrow where the incisions can be hidden in the hair-bearing portions of the eyebrows. It is again very important to design the pedicle of each flap wide enough to maintain the vascular viability of the tip. The advancement flap can usually be sutured into place using the method of halving, but occasionally bilateral symmetrical Von Burow's excisions will be required.

O-T and A-T flaps

An O-T flap can be created by extending the wound laterally at either side of the base of a circular defect, and then advancing the resultant flaps to cover the defect by meeting in the mid-line (Fig. 20.24). An A-T flap is created by similar incisions at the base of a triangular defect, advancing the flaps to the midline and suturing the wound in the shape of a 'T' (Fig. 20.25). Both of these advancement flaps have the advantage that the pedicles are broad based, and there is little risk of vascular impairment They are particularly useful along the vermilion border of the lip (Fig. 20.26), along a natural crease or fold such as the mental crease, at the junctions of the forehead and the eyebrow or at the frontal hairline.

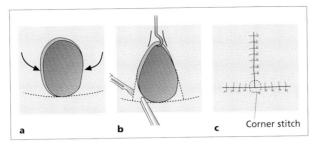

Fig. 20.24 O-T flap. **a.** Defect and design of advancement and **b.** flaps sutured in position.

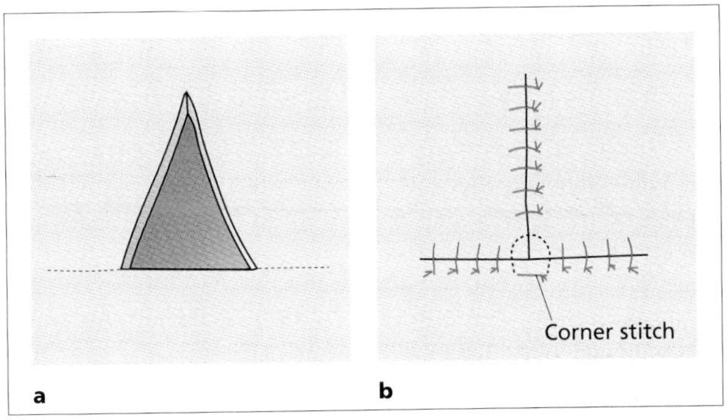

Fig. 20.25 A-T flap. **a.** Defect and design of flap and **b.** flaps sutured in position.

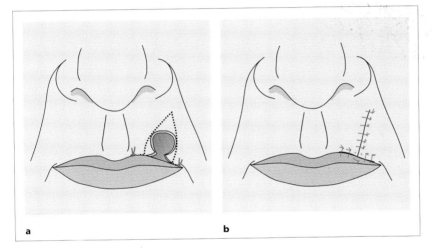

Fig. 20.26 A-T closure along vermilion border. **a.** Design of flap and **b.** flap sutured in position.

Subcutaneous island pedicle flap

This flap relies on the principle that the subcutaneous tissue is the most elastic component in the skin, thus tissue from the ends of an elliptical excision can be advanced, enabling closure of wounds with minimum tension using skin which would otherwise not be wanted. The flap creates a central island of skin, the blood supply being through the broad and deep vascularised fatty pedicle. This flap can be used on the limbs where two-island pedicles may be advanced from either end of the excision (Figs 20.27 & 20.28), or the cheek, where a single island pedicle may be used,

231

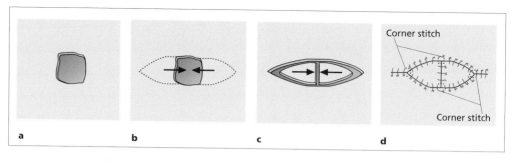

Fig. 20.27 Two-island subcutaneous pedicle flap. **a**. Defect; **b**. design of flaps for advancement; **c**. advancement of flaps; and **d**. flaps sutured in position.

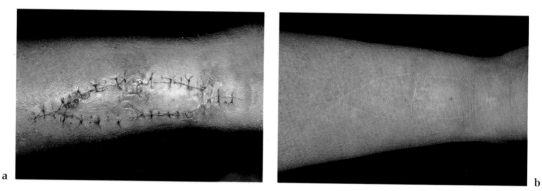

Fig. 20.28 Two-island subcutaneous pedicle flap on limb. **a**. Flap sutured in place and **b**. resultant scar at 3 months.

which takes advantage of the high vascular supply to the fat on the central cheek.

A variation of the island pedicle flap is the bilateral pedicle advancement flap, which is only suitable if the flap rests on a bed of deep fat, thus usually limiting its use to the central cheek. This flap depends on the creation of lateral fat pedicles which provide the blood supply, while the flap is undermined in the deep fat, thus permitting maximum mobility. The flap length must be planned such that it is long enough to reach the defect without creating tension, which may cause flap ischaemia.

For the creation of this flap, the skin is incised around the perimeter of the flap, initially just to, but not into, the fat. The apex of the flap is incised more deeply, thus increasing flap mobility. The whole flap is then mobilised at the deep level by gently advancing scissors through the original defect, and deeply undermining the fat beneath the flap, before advancing the scissors through the apex. Undermining should be carried out as deeply as possible to maintain a good blood supply, while considering which deep structures may be damaged. On the medial cheek, terminal branches of the facial nerve may be damaged without adverse effect, but on the lateral cheek the facial nerve may be damaged if dissection is not above the level of the fibrous fascia.

Mobility can then be further increased by superficial dissection laterally from the wound margins into the surrounding fat, thereby creating bilateral lateral subcutaneous fat pedicles. By advancing the flap into the defect using a skin hook, mobility and tension can be assessed, and tethering can be relieved by severance of any deep attachment; this creates more movement as compared to lateral dissection. The flap is then sutured in place.

Rotational flaps

Rotational flaps are random pattern flaps which use lateral tissue movement, with the flap rotating about a pivotal point. These flaps exploit tissue elasticity and permit large flaps to be raised, since rotational flaps usually have a broad base and therefore a good vascular viability.

O-Z closure

One of the simplest rotational flaps is the O-Z closure. This involves arcuate incisions from opposite poles of a circular defect, to create two small rotational flaps on either side of the defect (Fig. 20.29). These flaps are rotated into the defect and closed side by side (Fig. 20.30). This type of closure is particularly useful on limbs, and the anterior and posterior chest.

Rhomboid flap

The rhomboid flap is a particularly versatile flap and is shown in schematic form in Fig. 20.31. The defect is first fashioned into a rhombus with apical angles of 60° and 120°. An incision is extended perpendicularly from the apex of the 120° angle, the length of this incision being equal to the length of the other sides of the rhombus. Another incision of similar length is made at 60° from the end of the primary incision parallel to the side of the rhombus. The flap is then undermined, and transposed to close the primary defect; the transposition has the effect of also closing the secondary defect. A clinical example of use of the rhomboid flap is given in Fig. 20.32. This flap has the advantage of allowing a large number of possible lines of closure to be executed according to the presence of excess skin, skin tension lines and cosmetically important lines.

Nasolabial flap

The nasolabial flap is used to repair defects on the side of the nose and utilises excess tissue available from the medial cheek area (Figs 20.33 &

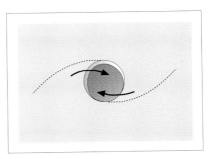

Fig. 20.29 Design of incisions for O-Z closure.

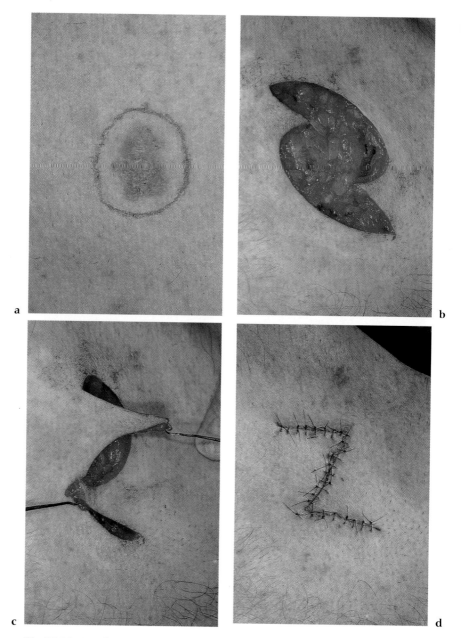

Fig. 20.30 O-Z closure. **a**. Initial lesion; **b**. wound after excision with arcuate incisions and undermining; **c**. flaps being pulled in place with skin hooks; and **d**. sutured Z closure.

20.34). The pedicle is superiorly based, with the secondary defect closed as a primary closure along the nasolabial fold. Incisions are made from the base of the defect along the nasolabial fold, and from the apex of this incision curving upwards. The flap is undermined, transposed by rotating it forwards and upwards, and then excess skin at the tip is trimmed off. The advantages of this flap include good colour and texture match, but the dis-

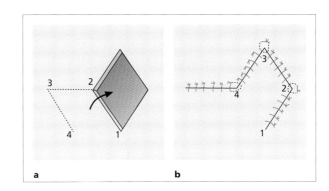

Fig. 20.31 Rhomboid flap.
a. Original defect and design of rhomboid rotational flap and **b**. rhomboid flap advanced and sutured in position.

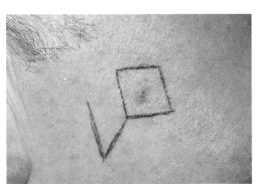

a

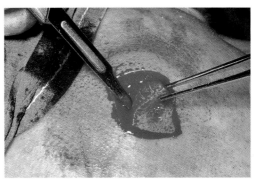

b

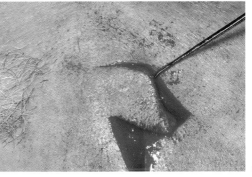

c

Fig. 20.32 Rhomboid flap. **a**. Design of rhomboid flap; **b**. excision of lesion; **c**. creation and advancement of flap; **d**. rhomboid flap sutured in position with corner stitches; and **e**. flap finally sutured in place.

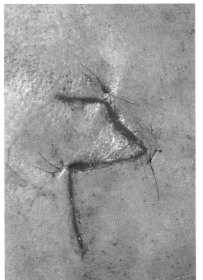

d

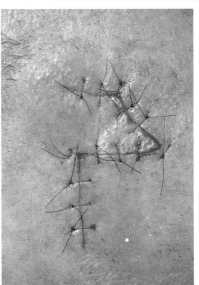

e

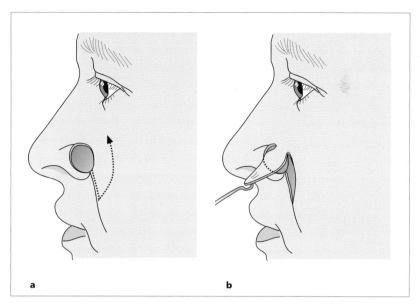

Fig. 20.33 Nasolabial flap. **a**. Design of nasolabial flap. **b**. Flap advanced and rotated to close defect; excess tip of flap needs to be excised.

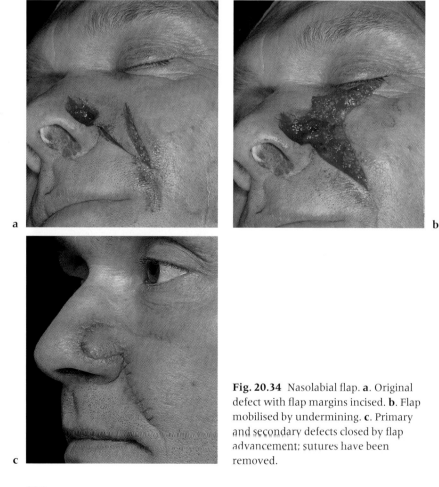

Fig. 20.34 Nasolabial flap. **a**. Original defect with flap margins incised. **b**. Flap mobilised by undermining. **c**. Primary and secondary defects closed by flap advancement; sutures have been removed.

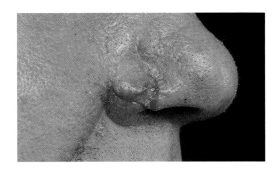

Fig. 20.35 'Trapdoor' deformity at apex of nasolabial flap 'dog-ear'.

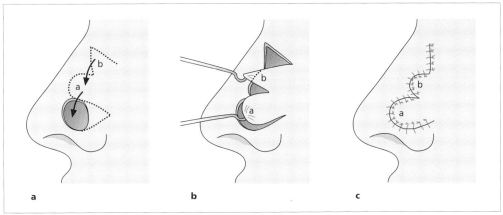

Fig. 20.36 Bilobed flap. **a**. Defect with design of flap; **b**. flap being rotated into position; **c**. flap trimmed and sutured into position.

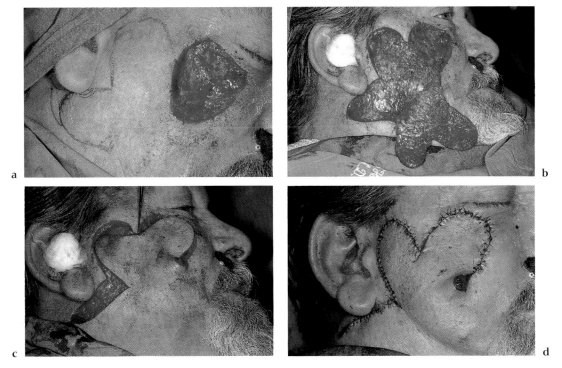

Fig. 20.37 Bilobed flap on cheek. **a**. Original defect with design of flap; **b**. mobilisation of flaps by undermining; **c**. advancement with rotation of flaps; and **d**. flaps sutured in position. 'Dog-ear' was repaired by curved removal away from flap pedicle.

advantage is that of a tendency to 'trapdoor' deformity, which may occur with contraction around the distal end of the flap (Fig. 20.35).

Bilobed flap

The bilobed flap (Figs 20.36 & 20.37) is particularly useful for the repair of defects on the nose; skin may be taken from the glabella for upper defects, or from the nasal side wall for lower defects. A modification of the bilobed flap has recently been described whereby the bilobed double transposition flap is accomplished with each flap rotating along an arc and transposed only 45°, with a Von Burow's triangle included in the initial design at the point of rotation.

20.11 Micrographic (Mohs') surgery

Mohs' micrographic surgery allows the controlled excision of infiltrative skin tumours by microscopic examination of horizontal sections cut from the periphery of an excision specimen, enabling maximal preservation of normal tissue but offering the best chance of tumour clearance. The method initially described by Mohs in the 1940s involved examination of tissue fixed *in vivo* and was thus a prolonged procedure extending over several days. This has now been almost entirely superseded by the fresh tissue technique, in which the lesion is excised and horizontal frozen sections are examined for residual tumour, thus usually enabling the procedure to be completed within 1 day. By precisely mapping residual tumour, it is possible to return to the exact anatomical location of remaining tumour strands, and to continue doing so until the tumour is completely extirpated. The technique is therefore much superior to the standard histopathological practise of 'bread-loaf' sectioning since, with the latter, residual tumour which happens to extend beyond the surgical excision margins at a site not sampled will be missed.

Mohs' micrographic surgery is indicated for tumours that spread by contiguous growth, such as basal cell carcinomas, but may fail in tumours that spread by satellitosis or exhibit skip areas, such as in melanoma or Merkel cell tumours. Basal cell carcinomas are the most common tumour treated by micrographic surgery; tumours that are large (greater than 1 cm), morphoeic, ill-defined tumours or tumour recurrences are all prime candidates for this technique (Fig. 20.38). Basal cell carcinoma has a propensity to follow the path of least resistance, and displays affinity for the fascial, perichondrial or peri-osteal planes, which makes tumour eradication difficult in sites such as around the temple, ala nasi, nasolabial regions, philtral ridge, peri-orbital region and peri-auricular areas; these are sites where Mohs' surgery may be used to greatest effect. It is also an important modality of treatment of basal cell carcinoma where perineural extension of the tumour is deemed likely.

Squamous cell carcinomas can similarly be treated in this way, especially at difficult anatomical sites that do not lend themselves to wide excision, or in the case of recurrent tumours. Other tumours treated with micrographic surgery include dermatofibrosarcoma protruberans, malignant fibrohistiocytoma, leiomyosarcoma and microcystic adnexal carcinoma. Sometimes,

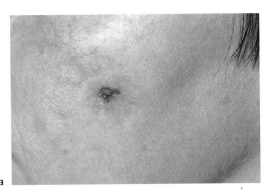
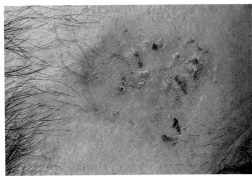

a

b

Fig. 20.38 Basal cell carcinomas suitable for Mohs' surgery. **a**. Morphoeic-type basal cell carcinoma; and **b**. ill-defined multicentric basal cell carcinoma.

there may be difficulty in interpreting frozen sections of these tumours, and in this case paraffin-embedded tissue sections, and/or use of monoclonal antibodies, may aid delineation of tumour strands from the surrounding tissues. There is controversy over the treatment of malignant melanoma by the micrographic technique because of the fear of missing satellites of tumour not contiguous with the primary tumour.

Technique

The stages of micrographic surgery are shown in Figs 20.39 and 20.40. The area that clinically appears to be involved with tumour is anaesthetised and the tumour debulked using a curette. The latter is important, as it reduces false positive results following tissue processing. A scalpel, angled at 45° to the skin, is then used to excise the tumour with a margin of normal looking epidermis; before the tissue is removed, the edges of both the specimen and the surrounding skin are notched (Fig. 20.40c), so as to enable exact tissue orientation throughout the process. A map is drawn, corresponding to the patient's defect (Fig. 20.40d), and the tissue is divided to create tissue segments that are small enough to be processed on a cryostat chuck (Fig. 20.40e). The borders of the tissue segments are stained with different colours of tissue dyes, to allow precise orientation of any tumour found on histopathology (Fig. 20.40f). Each segment is then turned over and compressed until flat. Horizontal frozen sections (5–7 μm) are then cut using a cryostat and stained. The horizontal sections taken from the underside of the segments include the whole of the excisional surface of this portion of skin, together with a thin rim of epidermis. If tumour deposits are noted on microscopy, further tissue is resected from the relevant area until a tumour-free plane is achieved (see Fig. 20.39). It is thus possible to remove only tumour-bearing tissue and to leave healthy tissue intact. Vital structures, such as part of the lacrymal apparatus, can often be retained, which would otherwise have had to been sacrificed to achieve tumour clearance when using a conventional surgical approach.

During the time when the tissue is being processed, the patient can wait with a simple dressing in place, and when tumour eradication has been achieved, the wound may be repaired appropriately or, alternatively,

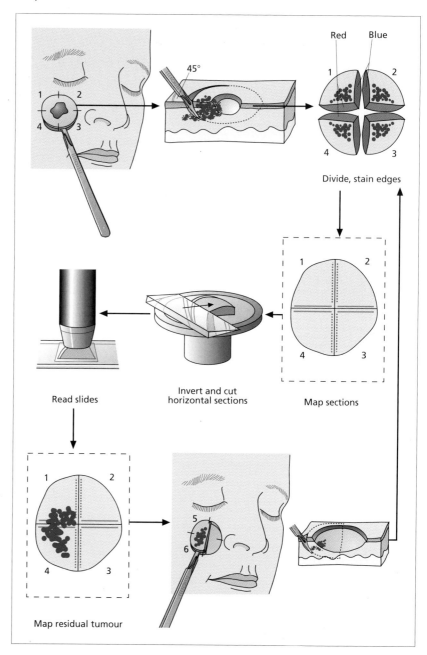

Fig. 20.39 Schematic summary of the stages of micrographic surgery.

allowed to heal by secondary intention. The decision on the mode of wound closure is often determined by patient preference, with younger healthy patients often wishing reconstructive surgery, while older and frail patients, who may not be fit for extensive surgery, often opt for secondary intention healing. If the reconstruction is very large, then myocutaneous flaps or more complex procedures can be carried out in collaboration with

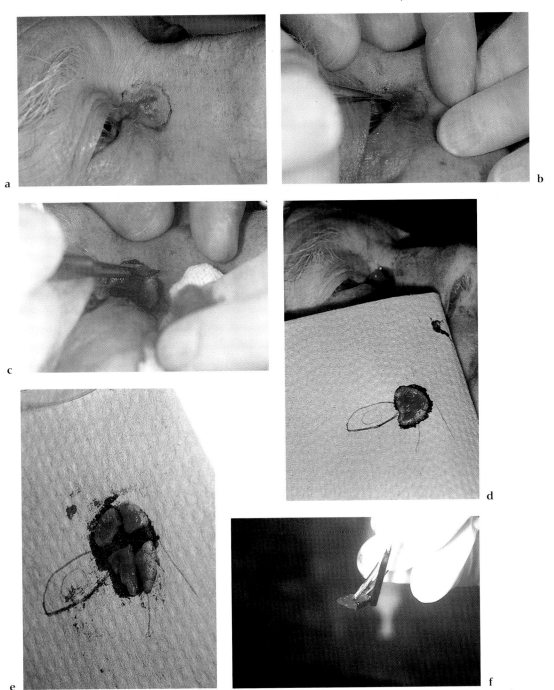

Fig. 20.40 Mohs' micrographic surgery. **a**. Original lesion; **b**. debulking with spoon curette; **c**. excision and notching; **d**. orientation of tissue maintained on free-drawn map; **e**. division of tissue in line with notches, maintaining anatomical orientation; **f**. inking of tissue segment edges for orientation.

241

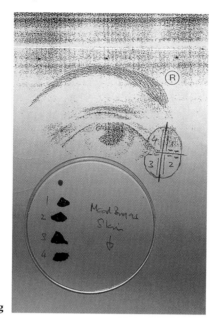
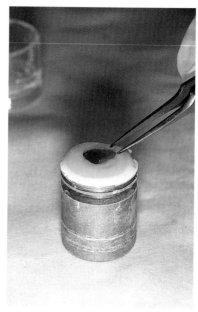

g

h

Fig. 20.40 *Continued* **g**. tissue ready for transport to laboratory together with map; and **h**. tissue inverted on cryostat chuck.

plastic, ophthalmic or faciomaxillary surgeons. Using the frozen tissue technique, even extensive lesions can often be excised in one session under local anaesthesia, without the necessity for hospital admission.

In some centres it may be difficult for frozen sections to be performed, or it may be decided that use of immunohistochemical techniques is required. In these circumstances, tissue can be processed for paraffin-embedded sections. This leads to a delay of 24–48 h, but often does give better histological definition of tissue structures, and enables inflammatory reactive changes and tumour cells to be differentiated more readily. The fixed tissue technique is probably best when dealing with tumours such as atypical fibroxanthoma, dermatofibrosarcoma protruberans and Merkel cell carcinoma. It has the disadvantage that reconstruction of the patient's wound may not proceed for several days, but studies have shown that this does not seem to increase the complication rate for reconstructive surgery. Paraffin-embedded tissue is usually also required if bone or cartilage are involved with tumour; with the former, the bony tissue will need to be decalcified, which considerably extends the processing time.

Micrographic surgery gives high cure rates, such as a 98–99% 5-year cure rate for basal cell carcinomas. Such high cure rates are particularly impressive when it is remembered that many of the tumours treated by micrographic surgery are the most difficult, or have already recurred on several occasions.

20.12 Laser surgery

A wide variety of lasers are now available for the treatment of cutaneous lesions. The therapeutic application depends on the wavelength, power density and energy. The choice of laser depends on the desired effect and the absorption characteristics of the target tissue. Only a brief summary will be given here.

Laser is an acronym for **l**ight **a**mplification by the **s**timulated **e**mission of **r**adiation. The key to laser use is the development of a monochromatic light source, enabling the beam to have an extremely high and precise power density. Ideally, for each particular clinical application, a laser should be chosen with exposure characteristics which provides selective photothermal damage of the target tissue, while sparing the surrounding tissue. For example, a flashlamp pumped dye laser tuned to a wavelength of 585 nm (yellow), an absorption peak of oxyhaemoglobin, and with an exposure time of 450 microseconds, is able to selectively damage small blood vessels and is therefore useful in the treatment of vascular lesions (Figs 20.41 and 20.42). The laser light is delivered via an optical fibre to hand pieces with spot sizes of 2–10 mm. High energy pulses immediately disrupt blood vessels but allow cooling (thermal relaxation) to occur such that heat diffusion into the surrounding tissue is insufficient to cause non-specific epidermal or dermal damage. Any risk of scarring is therefore minimised.

Types of laser

Carbon dioxide laser (10 600 nm)

This laser has a wavelength in the far infrared, which is rapidly absorbed by water and therefore body tissues. There is no selectivity in its effect. When a beam of carbon dioxide laser radiation strikes tissue, cells are vaporised instantaneously. Vaporisation is limited to cells immediately in the path of the beam, although there is a band of thermal damage around the treatment site. The width of this band depends on the power density and exposure time. The carbon dioxide laser is useful for tissue destruction of an extremely precise degree and may be used to treat a large variety of skin lesions including recalcitrant warts, epidermal naevi,

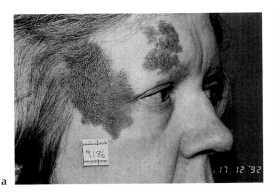
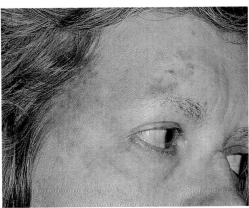

a

b

Fig. 20.41 Treatment of capillary haemangioma (port wine stain) with tunable dye laser. **a**. Original lesion and **b**. following therapy.

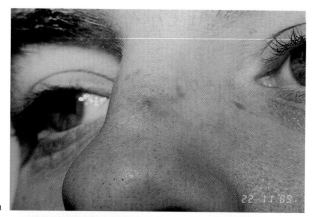

a

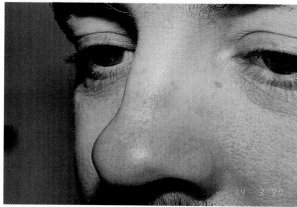

b

Fig. 20.42 Treatment of spider naevus with tunable dye laser. **a**. Original lesion and **b**. following therapy.

keloids, actinic cheilitis, rhinophyma and tumours. Many of its potential uses have been compromised in the past by unwanted thermal damage and consequent scarring. The recent development of accurate scanning systems has made the treatment of superficial lesions much more precise and broadened the application of the carbon dioxide laser in aesthetic surgery.

Research continues into newer systems, with absorption coefficients that may be more precise, and early reports of the clinical efficacy of the erbium-YAG laser (2940 nm) are promising.

Lasers for vascular lesions

Argon laser (488/514 nm)

This laser produces a blue/green light which is absorbed by melanin and haemoglobin. The therapeutic effect depends on the production of a coagulative necrosis and it was the first laser to be used to attempt to selectively treat vascular lesions. Whilst many of the early patients with capillary malformations derived benefit, there was a significant risk of scarring until the advent of accurate scanning systems. It is now used mainly to treat capillary malformations in adults. The argon laser and similar lasers such as the copper vapour (518/577 nm), the continuous wave dye laser (575 nm) and the frequency doubled neodymium-YAG laser (532 nm) are also extremely useful for treating fine telangiectasia, especially of the face, using a narrow incident beam (50–100 μm) to trace over and seal the vessels.

Pulsed dye laser (585 nm)

Dye lasers can be tuned to a selected wavelength and when pulsed can produce sufficient energy in a single short pulse to disrupt superficial dermal vessels with minimal damage to surrounding structures (see above). They are generally regarded as the treatment of choice for capillary malformations in children, capillary angiomas (when treatment is indicated), and other vascular lesions, particularly when extensive, uniform treatment is required, for example in widespread facial telangiectasia of poikiloderma of Civatte. In capillary malformations 90% of patients show lightening, with 50–75% improvement in the majority of patients after several treatments and 100% clearance in 10%. The incidence of texture change is <1%. There is a dramatic purpuric reaction which can be a problem when treating lesions for aesthetic reasons. Unfortunately, dilated superficial (thread) veins of the legs do not always respond, but a recently-developed non-coherent light source, the Photoderm® (515–1200 nm), is currently undergoing clinical trials; early results are promising in a variety of vascular lesions.

Lasers for pigmented lesions

The development of lasers which could selectively damage blood vessels led to a resurgence of interest in the possibility of using short pulsed, high energy lasers of appropriate wavelength to treat other 'coloured' structures in the skin.

'Q-switched' ruby laser (694 nm)

The red light from this laser is well absorbed by melanin and the blue/black ink of tattoos. High energy pulses cause the fragmentation of pigment clusters to smaller granules which can be taken up in phagocytic cells and removed via the lymphoreticular system. Treatment may often, as is the case with vascular lesions, be carried out without local anaesthetic, although topical, local or general anaesthetic can be used if necessary. Some pain and discomfort is felt during treatment but minimal post-treatment care is required with the area settling over a period of 2 weeks. The treated area fades over a few weeks when further treatment can be given. Several treatments are required, and complete removal cannot be assured.

There are also other lasers which have been developed for treating this type of condition and currently no single device will treat the entire range of clinical problems. Pulsed dye lasers (504 nm) can treat mainly superficial pigmented lesions. Alexandrite lasers (750 nm) and 'Q-switched' neodymium-YAG lasers (532 and 1064 nm) can both be used to treat pigmented lesions and tattoos. It is impossible to predict which laser system will produce the best result. Alexandrite lasers often prove useful for treating green colours and the neodymium-YAG laser at 532 nm often treats red inks effectively. Results in the treatment of a number of benign pigmented lesions are promising and further refinement of treatment protocols and laser systems will improve the outcome of treatment in many conditions.

Bibliography

Albright SD. Placing of 'guiding sutures' to counteract undesirable retraction of tissues in and around functionally and cosmetically important structures. *J Dermatol Surg Oncol* 1981; 7: 446–9.

Barlow RJ, Walker NPJ, Markey AC. Treatment of proliferative haemangiomas with the 585 nm pulsed dye laser. *Br J Dermatol* 1996; 134: 700–4.

Bennett RG. The meaning and significance of tissue margins. *Adv Dermatol* 1989; 4: 343–56.

Dinehart SM, Pollack SV. Metastases from squamous cell carcinoma of the skin and lip. *J Am Acad Dermatol* 1989; 21: 241–8.

Drake LA, Dinehart SM, Goltz RW *et al.* Guidelines of care for Mohs' micrographic surgery. *J Am Acad Dermatol* 1995; 33: 271–8.

Grabb WC. Skin grafts. In: Grabb WC, Smith JW, eds. *Plastic Surgery*, 3rd edn. Boston: Little, Brown, 1979: 16–35.

Grabb WC, Smith JE (eds). Basic techniques of plastic surgery. In: *Plastic Surgery*, 3rd edn. Boston: Little, Brown, 1979: 3–74.

Jackson IT. *Local Flaps in Head and Neck Reconstruction*. St Louis: CV Mosby, 1985.

Johnson TM, Sebastien TS, Lowe L *et al.* Carbon dioxide laser treatment of actinic cheilitis. *J Am Acad Dermatol* 1992; 27: 737–40.

Johnson TM, Ratner D, Nelson BR. Soft tissue reconstruction with skin grafting. *J Am Acad Dermatol* 1992; 27: 151–65.

Knabel MR, Koranda FC, Olejko TD. Surgical management of primary carcinomas of the lower lip. *J Dermatol Surg Oncol* 1982; 8: 979–84.

Land PG, Osguthorpe JD. Indications and limitations of Mohs' micrographic surgery. *Dermatol Clin* 1989; 7: 627–42.

Lang PG Jr. The partial closure. *J Dermatol Surg Oncol* 1985; 11: 966–9.

Lewis EL. A marsupialization procedure for repair of large cutaneous surgical wound. *Int J Dermatol* 1985; 24: 322–3.

Motley RJ, Holt PJA. The use of meshed advancement flaps in the treament of lesions of the lower leg. *J Dermatol Surg Oncol* 1990; 16: 346–8.

Petres J, Hundeiker M. Special techniques for different regions of the body. In: *Dermatosurgery*. Berlin: Springer-Verlag, 1978: 51–92.

Robins P, Dzubow LM, Rigel DS. Squamous-cell carcinoma treated by Mohs' surgery: an experience with 414 cases in a period of 15 years. *J Dermatol Surg Oncol* 1981; 7: 800–1.

Robinson JK. *Fundamentals of Skin Biopsy*. Chicago: Year Book Medical Publishers, 1986: 30–9.

Sebben JE. Wedge resection of the lip: minimizing problems. *J Dermatol Surg Oncol* 1985; 11: 60–4.

Spicer MS, Goldberg DJ. Lasers in dermatology. *J Am Acad Dermatol* 1996; 34: 1–25.

Swanson NA. Mohs' surgery. Technique, indications, applications and the future. *Arch Dermatol* 1983; 119: 761–73.

Swanson NA. *Atlas of Cutaneous Surgery*. Boston: Little, Brown, 1986.

Walker NPJ, Bailin PL. Dermatological surgery. In: Champion RH, ed. *Recent Advances in Dermatology*, Vol. 7. Edinburgh: Churchill Livingstone, 1986: 211–31.

Wheeland RG, Bailin PL, Ratz JL *et al.* Carbon dioxide laser vaporization and curettage in the treatment of large or multiple superficial basal cell carcinoma. *J Dermatol Surg Oncol* 1987; 13: 119–25.

21 Complications of dermatological surgery

Many complications of dermatological surgery can be prevented, or at least anticipated, from a thorough preoperative assessment of the patient. Patients with a bleeding diathesis or those on aspirin or anti-coagulants should be identified preoperatively; if possible, the coagulation profile should be corrected or the anti-coagulant should be stopped prior to surgery. If this is not possible, it may be worth considering other approaches to the patient's problem, such as radiotherapy, or postponing the procedure until such time as the patient's anti-coagulant can be safely stopped. Infection in surrounding tissues may be treated preoperatively using either topical or systemic antibiotics, thus reducing the possibility of wound infection following surgery. A history suggestive of allergy to antibiotics or dressings must be identified before surgery if potentially serious, yet entirely avoidable, complications are to be prevented. It is important to realise that many complications may be inter-related. A wound that has a haematoma is more likely to become infected and, in turn, both of these complications are likely to lead to wound dehiscence.

21.1 Haematoma

Perhaps the most common of all complications in dermatological surgery is that of bleeding and haematoma formation in the first postoperative days. Minor bleeding may follow the waning of adrenaline vasoconstriction, or result from hypertension or excessive wound movement. Another reason for excessive bleeding following surgery is the ingestion of aspirin or some other anti-inflammatory drug prior to surgery (Fig. 21.1). Aspirin can affect platelet aggregation for the lifetime of the platelet, and is therefore best withheld for 2 weeks before and 1 week after surgery. It is important to instruct patients to avoid aspirin, aspirin-containing compounds and non-steroidal anti-inflammatory drugs (NSAIDs). They should be advised to use paracetamol instead. Alcohol is also a potent vasodilator and is known to cause postoperative bleeding; patients should be asked to limit alcohol intake in the preoperative period. Patients should be instructed that, if bleeding does occur from the wound, firm direct pressure should be applied for 10–15 min; this will often bring bleeding from a superficial wound under control. Other precipitating events which can lead to haematoma include trauma to the wound area, and even minor motion such as in chewing or talking may increase bleeding in wounds close to the mouth.

Major bleeding is usually the result of inadequate intraoperative haemostasis or bleeding from vessels which were not noted during surgery. Haemostasis must therefore be meticulous and thorough during surgery. Larger vessels must be clamped and ligated with absorbable sutures, while smaller vessels may be sealed using electrosurgery. A bipolar device using

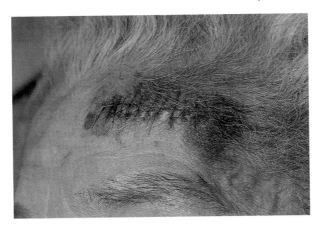

Fig. 21.1 Bruising and haematoma formation in a patient taking aspirin and systemic steroids.

low voltage and high frequency, thereby causing less tissue destruction, is to be preferred. Where this is not available, other modes of cautery are adequate, but it is unwise to use excessive cauterisation, as this will leave charred and necrotic tissue which predisposes to wound infection.

The earliest warnings of a haematoma will be of increasing pain or swelling in the area of the wound, which will subsequently become blue and tender. Patients must therefore be instructed to seek medical advice if their wound suddenly becomes painful. If this does occur, sutures should be removed as quickly as possible to decrease the tension on the wound and prevent further ischaemia and tissue damage. The clot should be completely evacuated and the wound irrigated with sterile saline, before dealing with the bleeding problem. A rolled piece of gauze or sponge may be used with a firm rolling motion to force the blood and clots to the wound opening. If this is done early the wound can be resutured, but since blood is an excellent medium for bacterial growth, it is usually wise to start the patient on an antibiotic prophylactically to prevent wound infection.

Occasionally, a haematoma that is not tender or expanding may be left and, after liquefaction of the clot at around 10 days, the serous fluid may be aspirated through a needle or through a stab wound made some distance from the wound edge, using a No. 11 scalpel blade.

21.2 Wound infection

A clean wound free of blood and tissue debris normally resists infection even in the presence of significant numbers of bacteria. It follows that much action can be taken during the operative procedure to reduce the risk of subsequent wound infection. The early signs of wound infection are those of increased erythema, swelling, pain and heat in the area of the wound. There may be evidence of tenderness in the surrounding tissue, and in more advanced cases lymphangitis in the surrounding tissue or a purulent exudate appearing from the wound. Infection of the wound usually becomes evident between the fourth and eighth postoperative day, and is most common in prolonged operations or on sites where there are larger numbers of resident bacteria such as on the perineum, axilla and ears. Wound infection is also more frequent in patients who are immunocompromised either through immunosuppressant or cytotoxic drugs including systemic corticosteroids, or as a result of malnutrition, diabetes or renal or hepatic failure. Wound infection is also increased by poor surgical technique, including excessive tissue destruction or necrosis, and foreign bodies in the wound (sutures, excessive diathermy, surgical drains).

If the signs of infection are noted early it is sometimes possible to treat with antibiotics and to leave the sutures in place and simply observe the wound, as would be the case with a stitch abscess. However, when the wound is grossly inflamed and fluctuant, and there is inflammatory oedema, the sutures must be removed and the wound irrigated with sterile saline. In this situation, the wound will usually have to be left open to heal by secondary intention with, if necessary, revision of the scar at a later stage. Wherever possible, the infecting organisms should be isolated by culture of pus or infected tissue and the patient commenced on the appropriate antibiotic as determined by bacterial sensitivities. Penicillin or erythromycin and flucloxacillin can usually be prescribed, if necessary, while sensitivity results are awaited. Wound infections are most commonly due to *Staphylococcus aureus*, with *Streptococcus pyogenes* being less common.

21.3 Wound dehiscence

Wound dehiscence (Fig. 21.2) may occur as a result of either systemic or local factors. Systemic factors which increase the likelihood of wound dehiscence include old age, diabetes, poor nutrition and systemic steroids. Local factors include forceful tissue movement, inappropriately weak sutures, poorly secured knots, closure under tension (Fig. 21.3), sutures that are too tight causing tissue necrosis, premature removal of sutures or sutures cutting through tissue because they have been placed too close to the wound margins. Wound dehiscence can be prevented to some extent by using skin suture tapes to support the wound edges following removal of sutures. Wound dehiscence typically occurs within 2 weeks of suture removal, and this is perhaps not that surprising considering that the wound will have regained only 3% of its original strength by this time and only 35% by 1 month.

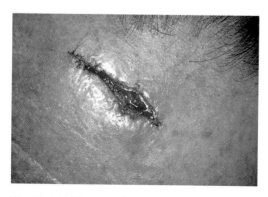

Fig. 21.2 Dehiscence of a sutured wound.

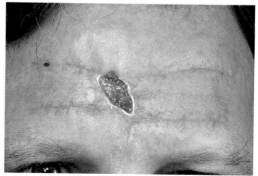

Fig. 21.3 Tip of flap necrosis due to closure under tension.

If dehiscence is encountered within the first 6 days and there is no evidence of wound infection, the wound may be resutured immediately. It is probably best not to excise the edges of such a wound, as fibroblastic activity will have already commenced and should be allowed to proceed.

21.4 Reaction to sutures

Sutures that are left in for longer than about 10 days can induce the formation of a foreign body reaction manifested by sterile pustules ('stitch abscesses') surrounding each of the sutures. This complication is most likely to occur on the chest, back, extremities and sebaceous areas of the face and settles following suture removal. Another complication is that of 'suture spitting', which describes the phenomenon of extrusion of subcutaneous sutures placed too high in the dermis, through the wound, usually without inflammation. Although worrying to the patient, this latter complication can be easily resolved by simple removal of the sutures.

Nodules in scars can develop around sutures on starch powder or talc (silicate) transferred from surgical gloves to the surface of the sutures, thus inducing a granulomatous foreign body reaction. Again, treatment may necessitate suture removal.

21.5 Contact dermatitis

Another cause of an acutely erythematous area surrounding a wound is that of contact dermatitis to a topical antibiotic or wound dressing. Such contact dermatitis is more common with antibiotic ointments, adhesive tape, tincture of benzoin or the surgical scrub solutions used for skin preparation. The patient may complain of pruritus, and in the extreme case there may be an intense bullous reaction, as with contact dermatitis to colophony in adhesive tape.

Treatment of this complication consists of the use of a topical steroid for a few days; this does not seem to have a deleterious effect on wound healing. It may be advisable to carry out patch testing in due course so that the patient can be advised of the allergy and avoid this complication in future.

21.6 Spread scar

There are few things more depressing than achieving a very good result at the time of suture removal only to see the patient some 6 months later to find that the scar has spread and, in the acute phase, is still red. This occurs most frequently on the upper chest, shoulders and back, where strong muscles create tension on the wound edges and may lead to a stretched scar (Fig. 21.4). This can, to some extent, be prevented by the use of subcutaneous sutures which remain in place for many months, providing wound support. Scar spreading can also be prevented by warning the patient, where possible, to limit excessive strain on the area until healing has strengthened the wound, which may take several months. On the back, excision of lesions followed by allowing the wound to heal by secondary intention can sometimes lead to a better cosmetic scar, with less spreading of the scar than occurs when a wound has been sutured. When a spread

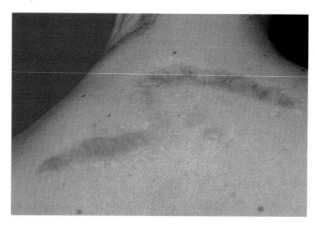

Fig. 21.4 Spread scar on back.

scar does occur, the initial redness will settle in 1 year to 18 months and the patient may be satisfied with this result. Otherwise, the scar will have to be excised and resutured with subcutaneous suture technique.

21.7 Keloids and hypertrophic scars

Keloid and hypertrophic scars are the result of increased fibroblastic activity within the scar. A keloid grows and extends beyond the boundaries of the original scar, whereas a hypertrophic scar is maintained within the boundaries of the injury and tends to widen with time. Hypertrophic scars seem to reach their peak in about 3 months and then tend to soften and regress, while keloids may increase in size for 6 months or more and may never regress.

Keloid reactions occur most frequently on the neck, shoulders, upper chest and back, and both keloids and hypertrophic scars probably occur more frequently in wounds that have been closed under tension. Keloidal reaction is much more common in black, Polynesian and Chinese people than in white populations and probably also occurs most frequently in young adults.

Intralesional steroid therapy is a very popular modality for treating keloid scars. Because of the variation in patient sensitivity to triamcinolone, it is best to start off with test doses of 10 mg/ml injected into the main bulk of the keloid and repeat once before increasing to 40 mg/ml. Repeat injections should not be undertaken in less than 8 weeks. The initial injection of intralesional steroid into keloids can be difficult and may be facilitated using pressure jet apparatus, cryotherapy to the keloid some 20 min before the injection to soften the keloid and induce oedema, and the use of a syringe and needle with a luer lock, so that the needle does not come adrift. Smaller keloids can at least be improved, although complete regression is not usual and recurrence has been described. This treatment is not without its problems, as it can induce overlying skin atrophy, perilesional linear skin atrophy, telangiectasia, depigmentation and ulceration.

The use of topical steroids, including Haelan® tape (fluorandrenolone impregnated into an adhesive tape), is unlikely to be of much therapeutic benefit unless the keloid is extremely thin, soft and new. Topical steroids may overcome the itch in a keloid.

Cryotherapy on its own, or in combination with intralesional steroid, has been used to treat keloids, but has the disadvantage of causing depigmentation, especially in pigmented skins. It probably works best in conjunction with intralesional steroid therapy, where objective improvement has been noted in up to 80% of cases.

Pressure has long been used as a treatment for keloid scarring with a variety of pressure garments being available. It can also be used to good effect following surgery in those who have a predisposition to keloids, in an attempt to stop keloid formation. Various devices have been described to treat earlobe keloid reactions, including a decorative spring-pressurised earring which can be left in place following surgical reduction of earlobe keloids for a few weeks. A synthetic polybutadine acrylate sponge held in place over the keloid by means of a pressure garment for 18–20 h/day for 6 months has been effective. Silicone gel pads or gel sheeting (Fig. 21.5) (Silastic®, Cica-Care®) held in place on the scar with a light dressing is also quite effective in some cases. This approach has been used on post-burn keloids, but is obviously only suitable where pressure garments can be worn.

Surgical excision of keloids usually leads to quick recurrence in 45–100% of cases, especially if efforts are not made to minimise tension, trauma and subcutaneous sutures in the wound. The recurrence rate can be decreased by either injection of the wound edges with corticosteroids during the early weeks and months, or by the use of radiotherapy using either external beam or yttrium implants to the wound edges, as soon as possible after surgery to decrease the fibroblastic response. Radiotherapy may, however, cause hyperpigmentation, telangiectasia and atrophy. Radiotherapy on its own has also been used in the treatment of keloids with response rates of 16–94%; the best response rates occur with relatively new keloids, while keloids are generally unresponsive if they are older than 6 months. Total doses of between 200 and 2000 cGy, administered over 1–2 weeks, have been recommended.

Newer treatments for keloids include excision with the carbon dioxide laser and allowing the area to heal by secondary intention, but it is doubtful

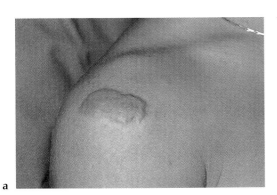
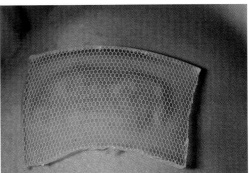

a   b

Fig. 21.5 a. Keloid on shoulder and **b**. with Silastic® gel plate in place.

if this produces superior results (39–92% recurrence rates) over conventional surgical techniques. Other treatments under investigation are topical tretinoin cream and interferon-α 2β, but further trials are necessary on these therapies before they can be routinely recommended.

21.8 Pigmentary problems

Pigmentary problems can sometimes follow dermatological surgery in those with dark skins. Patients must be warned of the possibility of hyperpigmentation or hypopigmentation in the scar before surgery. Hypopigmentation is common both in white and black skin following certain procedures such as dermabrasion, chemical peels and cryosurgery. Sunscreens may help to decrease pigmentary changes, and the latter may improve with time. In certain instances, such as following cryosurgery where melanocytes may be permanently damaged, there is little effective treatment that can be advised apart from cosmetic camouflage.

21.9 Nerve damage

One of the most serious complications of dermatological surgery is damage to cutaneous nerves, leading to loss of sensation or motor function. Mild numbness in the region of a scar is not uncommon due to the transection of small nerves, and in such cases the sensation can be expected to return after about 12–18 months, following regeneration of damaged sensory nerves. Numbness on the scalp is particularly common after deep resections on the forehead, following transection of nerves which course up the forehead onto the scalp. The return of sensation may be preceded by sensations of shooting pains, itching, crawling sensations and tenderness.

If, however, a large branch of a cutaneous nerve is severed it may not regenerate, leading to permanent loss of sensation and/or motor function. For example, if the temporal branch of the facial nerve is injured following surgery over the zygomatic arch there may be depression of the ipsilateral eyebrow, with an inability to wrinkle the forehead. This may require corrective surgery to overcome the effects of the nerve paralysis, and is the sort of damage that most often leads to costly medico-legal problems. Similarly, transection of the mandibular branch of the facial nerve results in drooping of the lip and asymmetry of the lip on movement. Division of the spinal accessory nerve in the posterior triangle of the neck results in shoulder drop, paraesthesiae and pain or difficulty in abduction of the arm.

The accidental division of a major nerve trunk should result in the patient having an attempted repair of the nerve by a plastic surgeon or neurosurgeon within 48 h, as undue delay prevents successful grafting of the nerve.

21.10 Ectropion

Every effort should be made to avoid the formation of an ectropion, which occurs especially in the elderly following lower eyelid surgery. Preoperatively, lesions of the lower lid should be assessed using the 'snap test' to examine lower lid laxity and the potential for ectropion formation. For

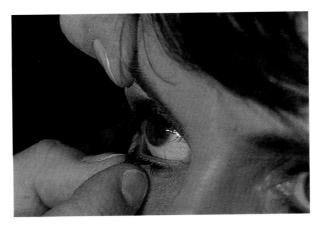

Fig. 21.6 'Snap test'.

this, the lower lid is grasped between the thumb and forefinger and is pulled away from the globe ('snap test'; Fig. 21.6). If the lid snaps back quickly, ectropion is less likely than if it only slowly returns to the surface of the globe. Great care must be taken to reduce the risk of an ectropion developing, and where a graft is necessary it should be 30% larger than the defect.

If the risk of ectropion seems high or when ectropion subsequently does occur then the assistance of an oculoplastic surgeon should be sought.

21.11 Persistent pain and pruritus

Pruritus is a common symptom in wound healing and at an early stage can be regarded as entirely normal. It can, however, be troublesome in some scars, and is particularly associated with keloid formation and in wounds that have been allowed to heal by secondary intention. This can often be settled with the use of a moisturiser such as topical Vaseline®, but if the problem becomes intractable, intralesional steroids may be required. Persistent pain in the region of the scar can occur in the form of neuritis when the scar tissue entraps a nerve. This can also be settled sometimes with intralesional steroids, but may require more elaborate treatment such as subcutaneous nerve stimulation or a more formal nerve block. Another cause of postoperative pain is the persistence of tumour within perineural nerve sheaths, in which case the pain is likely to be continuous. The surgeon may be alerted to this complication if histology reveals incomplete excision of a tumour.

Bibliography

Ahn ST, Monafo WW, Mustoe TA. Topical silicone gel for the prevention and treatment of hypertrophic scar. *Arch Surg* 1991; 126: 499–504.

Beard C. Eyelid skin surgery. In: Epstein E, Epstein E, eds. *Skin Surgery*, 6th edn. Philadelphia: WB Saunders, 1987: 482–91.

Berman B, Bieley HC. Keloids. *J Am Acad Dermatol* 1995; 33: 117–23.

Halvorson GD, Halvorson JE, Iserson KV. Abscess incision and drainage in the emergency department. *J Emerg Med* 1985; 3: 227–32.

Harahap M. *Complications of Dermatological Surgery. Prevention and Treatment.* Berlin: Springer-Verlag, 1993.

Meythiaz AM, de Mey A, Lejour M. Treatment of keloids by excision and postoperative radiotherapy. *Eur J Plast Surg* 1992; 15: 13–16.

Murray JC. Keloids: a review. *J Am Acad Dermatol* 1981; 4: 461–70.

Quinn KJ. Silicone gel in scar treatment. *Burns* 1987; 13: S33-S40.

Salasche SJ. Acute surgical complications: cause, prevention, and treament. *J Am Acad Dermatol* 1986; 15: 1163–85.

Salasche SJ, Bernstein G, Senkarik M. In: *Surgical Anatomy of the Skin.* Connecticut: Appleton and Lange, 1988.

Sproat JE, Dalcin A, Weitauer N, Roberts RS. Hypertrophic sternal scars: silicone gel sheet versus Kenalog injection treatment. *Plast Reconstr Surg* 1992; 90: 988–92.

Index

Page references in *italics* refer to illustrations; those in **bold** refer to tables.